First, You Cry

··

BETTY ROLLIN

···

First, You Cry

J. B. Lippincott Company
Philadelphia and New York

U.S. Library of Congress Cataloging in Publication Data

Rollin, Betty.
  First, you cry.

  1. Breast—Cancer—Personal narratives. 2. Rollin,
Betty. I. Title.
RC280.B8R64   616.9'94'490926   76–16047
ISBN–0–397–01167–9

*For my spirited, smart,
and loving mother*

Author's Note

I wish to thank Gerald Walker, who was the first to say, "Why don't you do a book about it?"; Genevieve Young, my editor, whose taste, brains, and sense of humor made the book better at every turn; and Allene Talmey, for giving me the benefit of her sharp eye.

And I especially want to thank M. Z., who saw the book through its birth, nurtured it, and shared its pleasure and pain.

On September 30, 1974, an NBC News correspondent reporting from the Guttman Breast Diagnostic Institute in New York told of the nationwide reaction to the mastectomy of the wife of the President of the United States—how women everywhere were rushing to their nearest mammographer, how suddenly afraid women were. The report emphasized that the fear was productive, because so many women were acting on it.

On camera, the correspondent said, "The terror that women feel about breast cancer is not unreasonable. What is unreasonable is that women still turn their terror inward. They think if they avoid investigating the possibility that they have the disease, they'll avoid the disease. But as cases of such prominent women as Betty Ford become known, other women are turning their fear into the kind of action that can save their lives."

The correspondent had done her homework. She knew that early detection was important, that most lumps were benign. She knew all about the different kinds of mastectomies—radical, simple, and so on—and the controversies about them. She knew a lot. But as the correspondent spoke to the camera, telling the nation what she knew about breast cancer, there was one thing she did not know. She did not know that she had it herself.

First, You Cry

1

I HAD A LUMP for a year. At least a year. It was a hard little thing—about the size of a yellow grape—and it resided, imperceptible except to the touch, on the far left side of my left breast, due west of the nipple. I knew it was there, my (ex-)husband knew it was there, my (ex-)internist knew it was there, and my (ex-)mammographer knew it was there. Of the four, only one of us was worried about it. That was Arthur Herzog, the husband, who had found it on a spring evening in 1974 during a routine sexual feel.

"What's that?" he said. "I don't know," I said. "It's a lump," he said. "Mmmm," I said, wanting to sleep. "Will you get it looked at?" he said. "Sure," I said, and went to sleep.

I got it looked at. "It's nothing to worry about," said my internist on Central Park West, whom I'll call Dr. Smith. "Feels like a cyst. A lot of women have them. But we'll send you for some mammograms."

I went for some mammograms. "This doesn't worry me a bit," said my mammographer on East

Ninetieth Street, whom I'll call Dr. Ellby. He held up his pictures of my lump to the light. "Come back in a year and we'll have another look."

Whew. Not that I had been worried, either. Well, maybe just a little. Anyway, I was glad to be out of there.

Mammograms—low-radiation X rays that show the inner structure of the breast and can, theoretically, pinpoint the location of even the smallest abnormality—are not pleasant things to have. The experience is often likened to having a chest X ray, but it's not like that at all. When you have a chest X ray, you stand, shoulders forward, against a machine, and the machine performs. Mammograms require a different kind of participation. Before the picture-taking even begins, one has to tolerate the sensible and essential but unnerving business of being "palpated" (medically felt up) by the mammographer. Then, holding your paper gown together with one hand and grabbing your purse, bra, and blouse with the other, you are bustled off to another room where, topless and chilly, you sit on a small stool before a large machine. A technician— a young woman, usually, who moves fast and doesn't talk much—takes your breast in her hand and puts it, as if it were a slab of beef, on a slab of steel. Then her arm shoots up and she cranks down another slab of steel, thereby creating a sort of breast sandwich. Your flattened breast is the filling. "Say when it hurts," says the young woman, who has become part of the machine. "Ouch," you say, and she stops cranking. "Don't breathe," she says, as if you could. *Bam, slam. Click, slam.* "Breathe," she says. Then, like ballet exercises, repeat on the other side. (*Crank, crank.* "Don't breathe." *Bam, slam. Click, slam.* "Breathe.") And that's it. But you can't go home. Not yet. You go out to the waiting room filled with women on mahogany chairs and aqua settees reading *House Beautiful*s and old *Newsweek*s or not reading at all, and there you wait—either to be dismissed (no cancer) or called back for more pictures (maybe cancer). Not that that word is spoken either out here or in there. It is as silent as the *g* in *sign*. But, like the *g* in *sign,* it is there.

It was there in my head as I waited in Ellby's dreary waiting room on that day in June. But it was there the way "rape" was there. A buried terror, far, far under the ground.

My remote fear of breast cancer virtually ended when Ellby said he wasn't worried, and the fear was entirely finished off a week later when, after seeing the mammograms, Smith said *he* wasn't worried. Ellby was the mammogram emperor of the greater New York area ("Surgeons send their wives to him," a doctor friend had told me); Dr. Smith was my trusted (impeccably reputed) internist of eight years. If they weren't worried, why should I be?

"Don't be *silly!*" I barked at Arthur when he brought it up again a month later. "It's *nothing!* I had it looked at, didn't I?"

"But it's so hard," he said meekly.

"It's *supposed* to be hard. It's a fi-bro-ad-e-no-ma," I said, pronouncing each syllable, pleased with myself for remembering what it was called. "It's a cyst. Cysts are hard. A lot of women have them, and they're *not* cancer."

2

FOR ALMOST A YEAR, that was that. Although I did not worry about the lump, I could not entirely forget about it, either. It was, after all, there. Once in a while I'd feel it—sort of push it in with my index finger. It was an absentminded gesture, the way one feels a mole or a callus. Still there? Still there. Oh, well, isn't it nice that it doesn't mean anything.

When I did the breast cancer piece at the Guttman Institute, I remembered my lump as I interviewed one of the doctors, and considered asking one of them to have a look. No, that's silly. First of all, they're too busy. (I knew they'd squeeze me in, but I hated to ask.) And second, *I'm* too busy. The piece was to go on the air that night, which meant all the filming and the editing and the writing had to be done before five—and it was almost two. Besides, I reminded myself, two reputable doctors said it was nothing. So don't be a worrywart. Don't be a Jewish Princess. And, I scolded myself further, don't be a freebie-taker. Just because you're doing a story on a pastry shop doesn't mean you have to eat one of their Napoleons. To even contemplate mammogram payola seemed very low, indeed.

Besides, piped up my unconscious, you're a reporter. You're immune. You're doing a story about women with a possible affliction, you're not one of them. You're—the word is "covering" them—on the outside. You're a journalist. You've got credentials, press passes to get into places, or out. You can get assistance when you need it, or protection, if you need that. You're special. You're safe. You note screams in your spiral notebook, but they never come from your own throat.

It was not only my identity as a journalist that made me feel immune to disaster. There was also the fact of my past perfect health and, therefore, my identity as a perfectly, immutably healthy person.

I was always superbly healthy. My mother, true to the stereotype of Jewish mothers, used to make me eat. But, unlike the stereotype, she shoveled sirloin and wheat germ into the mouth of her baby girl, not matzoh brei or fatty chicken soup. When it came to food, Mother's rabbi was Carlton Fredericks, her guru Adelle Davis. My mother's kitchen never housed a potato chip or a slice of white bread. Once in a while, I had a hot dog at another child's birthday party. Usually, guilt would make me confess the transgression. "You ate that junk?" my mother would say. Then she would shake her head as if I were reporting a pregnancy, wondering where she went wrong.

One rebels against such a mother. I rebelled against mine. I smoked cigarettes and I had affairs with Christians. But I never ate a Baby Ruth or drank a Coca-Cola.

It must have worked. Both sides of the family were physical wrecks. But we Rollins—my father was subject to the same regimen—were beacons of good health. My mother took pride in my father's and my fitness the way other mothers took pride in their family's talent or good looks. And she loved to tell about what a mess my father was when he ate *his* mother's cooking. "She was a wonderful woman," my mother would say of my Russian grandmother. "But the way she cooked, it's a wonder she didn't kill her children."

Mother's food did not keep me from getting the usual childhood diseases, but I always had *mild* cases of everything, and I did seem to recover faster than other children struck with the same ailment. Needless to say, those facts did not go unnoticed by my mother. "It was such a little swelling, the doctor wasn't even sure it was mumps," she'd say to her sister on the phone. And "Have you ever heard of a child who had chicken pox for only three days?"

My mother's bragging about my constitutional superiority did not end with my childhood. "Betty never even takes aspirin," she said to Arthur once, before we were married. "She never even gets a *headache.*"

We giggled about it, afterward. "I never really worried that you were a dope addict," Arthur said. "Besides, I think you *ought* to get a headache once in a while. Who the hell wants to marry Wonder Woman?"

But I did not oblige. My mother, bore that she was on the subject, was right. I never did take aspirin. I almost never did get a headache. It crossed my mind that, notwithstanding the purity of my nutritional intake, I might be in for one of the family diseases. All the wheat germ in Kansas, I knew, might not protect me from inheriting gallstones, migraines, weak kidneys, or high blood pressure. But thirty-nine years of my life had passed and there was no sign of any of those afflictions, either. I never had so much as a passing worry about contracting a disease that was *not* in the family. As far as I knew, no one, living or dead, on my mother's side of the family or my father's, ever had cancer.

Almost a year passed. By now, due to the publicized mastectomies of Betty Ford and Happy Rockefeller, breast cancer was in the news. Because of that and because of my own piece, I knew a lot more about breast cancer than I had ten months ago. So did most people. Publicity educates, and so does fear. People were suddenly aware of the high incidence of the disease. Ninety thousand cases had been reported in 1974 alone. MORE WOMEN DIE OF BREAST CANCER, read a headline in *The New York Times*. "In North America and Western Europe one woman in twenty-five dies of breast cancer. In women in the twenty-five to thirty-four age group, the disease is second only to accidents and suicide

18

as a cause of death, while it is the leading cause for women aged thirty-five to fifty-four and, at higher ages, second only to cardiovascular diseases."

The question was, where did breast cancer come from? No one knew, but there were a lot of interesting guesses. Most of them were based on studies of who is most likely to get the disease: women with sisters, mothers, and aunts who had it; women who have not had children or who had them after the age of twenty; postmenopausal women; first-generation Jewish women of Eastern European ancestry; women with hypertension and diabetes. Then there was the virus theory, and the pill theory (never proved—they only know that female sex hormones are involved, somehow), and the animal fat theory (persuasive because of a huge study that showed that Japanese women who lived in America—and ate animal fats—tended to get breast cancer more than Japanese women who lived in Japan).

The frequency of the disease, accompanied by the jumble of inconclusive information about its possible causes, made a lot of women nervous and they began the rush to their nearest mammographers. The more they rushed, the more the press covered them rushing (as I had done); and the publicity, in turn, made other women rush. Women also learned how to examine their own breasts for lumps and did so frequently and frenetically. The message had definitely gotten through: Early detection may save your life.

19

Of course, fear did not always lead to action. Some women found lumps, themselves, but instead of doing something about it they became paralyzed with fear. "It's really a shame," someone from the American Cancer Society said to me on the phone one day. "Some of these women are killing themselves, and most of them really have nothing to fear. They think having a lump means they have cancer, and that's not true. Nine out of ten lumps are benign."

"I know that," I said to her. "As a matter of fact, I have one of those, myself."

3

I WENT BACK to Dr. Ellby before the year was up.
My first visit had been in June, 1974. Now it was
late March, 1975. The waiting room looked the
same: the same faded settees, the same pack of
women with the same range of facial expressions,
from bored to grim. Stupidly, I had forgotten to
bring something to read, so I was stuck with the
same old *House Beautifuls*.

After a half hour of "Remodeling Your Country
House" (I had none) and cute things to do with
shelf paper, I got angry. "How much longer?" I
asked the receptionist.

"It shouldn't be too much longer," she said,
lying.

Another half hour passed. There were about fifteen women in the waiting room now. Goddammit,
I thought, my feminist bile rising, they don't do
this to men. They wouldn't *think* of summoning
fifteen *men* all at the same bloody time in the middle of the bloody afternoon. Men have jobs; their
time is too valuable. They still think women don't
have anything better to do. Goddammit, at least the

bastard could get some decent magazines. "There is," I said with extreme hauteur to the flat-faced receptionist, whose eyeglasses were held together with a safety pin, "something wrong with your system." She gave me an I-only-work-here shrug. I went back to shelf paper.

Finally I was summoned. "Betty Rollin," said a nurse (pronouncing it Rowland) with a manila folder under her arm. I went in. Same rigmarole as last time. Strip to the waist. A little cursory feel from Dr. Ellby.

"That's my lump," I said when he got to it. He looked at me. "I had it a year ago. You said it was nothing and that I should come back in a year." I was annoyed at having to explain.

He nodded and drew a black circle around the lump with a pen. "That'll wash off," he said and walked out.

"Pick up your things and come with me, please," said the technician, young, small, and pale like last year's. Another breast sandwich, just as unpleasant. Besides, I was cranky. It was six o'clock. I had wasted an hour and a half so far.

I got dressed and went outside, took a walk around the block, and called my husband from the delicatessen on the corner. "I have to wait for the goddam pictures to be developed," I told him, "so it'll be at least another half hour."

I went outside and saw a pair of sandals in a store window that I thought were nice but didn't need.

I bought them. Outside, it had gotten colder. It looked like rain. I went back to Dr. Ellby's. When I got there, there were only two women left and the receptionist.

"He wants to do a few more," she said.

"Oh?" I said, and went in. This time Dr. Ellby himself did the job. No simple sandwich this time. Nor was it the same machine. This one was smaller (and colder) and instead of clamping the breast top and bottom, I had to bend over so he could clamp it together from the side. The problem, I gathered from his mumblings, was the location of the lump. It was so far over on the side that the other machine didn't get it. The pictures showed nothing bad; they just didn't show anything. All the same, I felt a small knot in my stomach.

"Uh, when do I get the results?" I said, trying not to sound worried.

"I'm going to Argentina Saturday," he began. (This was Thursday.) What the hell do I care where you're going? I thought. What a time to country-drop. What a creep. "Results will go in the mail . . ." blah blah . . . "Of course, if there's anything wrong, we'll call your doctor."

"When?"

"Tomorrow."

I had a pile of work to do the next day, in part because of the time lost (I still thought of it that way) *chez* Ellby. There was a piece to edit about *Ms.* magazine, which bored me, and another piece to research and set up on alcoholic teenagers, which didn't bore me at all. Someone who worked with young alcoholics in California had more or less promised that he could get me and a crew into a teenage Alcoholics Anonymous meeting out there, somewhere in the San Fernando Valley. That a teen AA group existed was astonishing, but in television something exists only if you can show it. Getting in to film that meeting, I knew, would make the story. The problem was I couldn't reach the man. I left messages all over the place, and I still hadn't heard back. Originally, he had said that there would be a meeting on the Monday coming up (it was now Friday), so that would mean going to the coast over the weekend, maybe even the next day.

Arthur and I had a dinner party planned for Saturday night. If the California trip worked out, we would have to call everybody up to cancel. Eleven thirty, the clock said. Dammit, I thought, I hate waiting for phones to ring. It's like being seventeen again, and anxious about Saturday night. I jiggled my pencil, I sighed, I thought about doing some work on the *Ms.* piece, couldn't face that, sighed again, and with the eraser end of the pencil punched another telephone line.

I called my mother about where to meet for our lunch date; I called the hairdresser for an appointment on Saturday in case I wouldn't be going to California. Then, when the other line *still* didn't ring, I flipped the Rolodex to Dr. Smith's number, stared at it for about ten seconds, and decided to let myself be a pest.

"I'm sorry to bother you," I said when he came to the phone, "but I was at Ellby's yesterday, and he said if anything were wrong, he'd call you, so I guess he hasn't, but I just thought I'd check because I'm probably going out of town. . . ."

He did not speak immediately, and when he spoke he pronounced each word as if he had had a rehearsal. The words I remember were " . . . nothing to worry about, but it really should come out."

I didn't speak right away, either. "When?"

"I'll give you the number of a surgeon, Dr. Singermann—he's first-rate. Make an appointment with him and he'll do the rest."

"Does it have to be right away?" I was vaguely alarmed, but mostly it sounded like another annoyance, more time wasted—as if the Dr. Ellby business weren't enough. Still, I wasn't expecting this. "I'm going to California for a week. Is it—should I try to get back sooner—I mean, how serious is it?"

"The end of the week would be just fine, Betty," said Dr. Smith, not really answering my question. "Look," he added, when he realized I was hanging on for more, "most of these things are benign. It just seems like a good idea to have it out. OK?"

OK? Sure OK. What choice did I have, not OK? I hung up and looked at the phone, but I was not thinking about California now. I was thinking about cancer. Not that I knew what to think. So I thought about the word. I said it to myself: Cancer. Then I thought about the lump, and then about the breast. My breast. I rubbed against it with the inside of my upper arm. Then the California call came through. Everything was arranged, said the man. We were in.

There, I thought, that's the life I know. Attaboy, life, *good* dog. See? Everything still works out for Betty. Nothing has changed. Not really. This is just a nuisance interruption. Annoying but necessary, like the time I had my wisdom tooth pulled and had to miss a friend's wedding. And looking back, it hadn't been such a long interruption. Having a lump removed doesn't take long, either, I thought. It can't be more than a day.

All the same, I called the surgeon from California. His secretary explained that it would be a good idea to book the hospital time now, as well as the office appointment preceding surgery. "Fine," I said. "How soon can it be?" The California story wouldn't take more than a few days. "How about next week?"

"Oh, no," said the secretary right away. "The appointment with the doctor is no problem, but I doubt if I can get you into the hospital before a few weeks at least."

"Would you try?" I said, wanting very much now

to have it over with. I bit off a piece of cuticle on my index finger and it started to bleed.

There was an odd pause. Then: "May I ask you something?" said the secretary. Then: "Are you on television?"

I smiled. "Yes," I said, aware in the same instant both that I had a trump card and that I would use it. From my short experience (as a fourth-string celebrity) I knew that because the secretary had seen me on television, she would probably make a special effort to get me into the hospital. It's hard to understand this sort of thing when there's nothing in it for the other person. But there it is.

Sure enough, an hour later, when I called back, it was all arranged. I would go into the hospital next Sunday, surgery would be Monday morning, and the Friday before, I would go to the office and see Dr. Singermann. It was appalling, of course, that just because the secretary happened to watch NBC News, I got a bed. All the worse, I suppose, because I was willing to take it. But I had my own code about these things: If the goods or privileges in the offing are not of serious or compromising value, and if I want whatever it is a lot (which I almost never do), I feel slightly queasy and take it. If I don't want whatever it is a lot, like getting the mammograms that day at the Guttman Institute, I feel slightly queasy and *don't* take it.

I made the second call from Millicent Braverman's house in Beverly Hills. Millie is an old friend who owns and runs an advertising agency. She is a big-boned, handsome woman, good-natured and very, very smart. She had had a lump taken out of her breast a year ago. It was benign. When I hung up on the call to New York, I must have looked less than tranquil. She shook her head and, to my surprise, started unbuttoning her blouse. "For Chrissake," she said, "I want you to see this. It's absolutely *nothing*." She yanked her breast out of her bra as if it were a book she thought I should read and with her other hand pointed at a small horizontal scar about an inch above the nipple. "Look," she commanded. "Nothing! And before it happened, I was scared *shitless*."

I laughed. "You're right," I said, trying to please her. "It really *is* nothing."

We both knew, of course, that what scared me—what had scared her—was not the scar from the removal of a benign breast tumor but what would happen if it were the other kind. In spite of my jitters, I also "knew" that, like my friend, I had a benign tumor. I, too, would have a little scar on my breast—but it would be on the side, so it would be even less noticeable.

It was nice, what Millie had done. If I ever knew anyone else who was about to have the operation, I thought, I'll be a pal and do the same for them. I'll show them my scar, the way Millie showed me hers.

In that brief, pseudo-altruistic fantasy, I had no particular victim in mind. The assumption, indeed the point of the fantasy, was that there was another victim, not me—someone else to whom this would happen. Someone else. Not me.

Later, months later, I wondered how I could have been quite so pigheadedly unafraid. It was as if there were a piece of embroidery in my head, reading: Bad Things Don't Happen to Me. Implanted at birth—as the only child of grateful, adoring parents, I always felt special and intrinsically protected from harm—the embroidery had more or less held up. Oh, there had been some dark days, especially in my twenties, when I didn't know what I wanted or how to get it. I suffered over men, like most women, agonized occasionally over work, and at one point I was miserable enough to get analyzed. (I was also rich enough to afford it.) Nor was I the kind of overprivileged only child who is merely smothered with love. I was smothered with love, but I was also prodded with expectation. I had everything, but I was expected to do something with it.

This is not the lot of all Jewish Princesses. Some, I know, are taken to Bonwit Teller a lot and expected to marry, period. But I was the Princess *and* the Prince. My parents were not disappointed when they had a girl instead of a boy. Why should they have been? With me, in effect, they had both. They expected me to marry (thank God she is pretty) *and* they expected me to be a doctor (thank God she is smart). Not a doctor, really; that would have been too odd. But I had to be Something.

That was okay with me. I wanted to be Something, too. Especially when I got older and found out that not being Something meant having a boring job or getting married so as not to have a boring job. (These were the late fifties, remember, when nice young women only worked *until* they got married.)

By a fluke, I became an actress. An agent had seen me in a college play—at Sarah Lawrence—sent me for an audition, and the day of my graduation I went into rehearsals off-Broadway as Miss Dainty Fidget in *The Country Wife*. It was fun. I didn't have much to say, but I hung about onstage, fanning myself with a feather. There is nothing lofty about being an actress in New York, but it was better than being a secretary. And, although I didn't become a star, I worked. And although the daily business of being an actress was often shoddy and painful, learning the craft of acting in professional classes (with Sanford Meisner and, later, Lee Strasberg) was as engrossing and enriching as anything I had ever done.

Then I slid into writing—first by selling a book idea to Doubleday, then by going on to other small books and magazine articles, bluffing my way into a job as a features editor at *Vogue,* and winding up, finally, at *Look* as a senior editor, with a column of my own.

I cared about my work, and when you care about something you are bound to get hurt some. But what small hurts they were. For the most part, I had a golden life, and like most people with golden lives, I took mine for granted. I was happy and smug. I had fulfilled society's expectations, my mother's, and, as I got analyzed and older, my own as well. I married late, but I married. I didn't have children, but I didn't want children. I cried when *Look* died, where I had been almost continuously euphoric, but then—having had the good sense not to run to *Life* (which died a year later)—I engineered myself into a fine job at NBC News. It was hard there at first, because I was hired to do something I didn't know how to do: be a news correspondent. Before NBC, I had had no experience either in hard news or in film producing (which is how news stories are covered). But I learned. I even got good at it.

Everything always worked out. I expected it to. Perhaps that's why it did. My talents were no greater than those of other people for whom things don't work out. But I was confident and lucky. My confidence, moreover, was not limited to myself but encompassed my world. I knew in my head that life was capricious and worse; I had read about the Nazi holocaust, I had a sense of what was going on in remote places like Vietnam and around the corner in Harlem. But—I couldn't help it—none of the bad stuff had ever touched me directly. In my life, deprivation, injustice, disease were as remote as Bangladesh . . . as unlikely as cancer.

4

ON FRIDAY, I was back in New York, in the Nightly
News film editing room. The film from the AA
meeting was terrific. What makes film terrific is
when the talkers—in this case, alcoholic kids—say
what is on their minds, as opposed to what would
either "sound good" or "be safe to say" for television. It helps if what is on their minds is interesting. And kids talking about becoming drunks at
fifteen and what happens next was riveting. I knew
if the AA film worked—and it did—it would tell the
story better than any expert I could find to describe
the problem.

When something works on film, there's a nice
kind of excitement in the editing room. We sat there
most of the day, the editor, the field producer, and
I, watching the film in the half-darkness, stopping,
starting, noting the parts that were especially good,
trying to figure out, as we went along, the order of
the story. Would it be best to start out on the AA
meeting? No, better save that for the end and begin
with film we had of kids drinking in a bar upstate.
Lay out the problem first, then go from there.

I had scheduled the appointment with Dr. Singermann late in the day, so that it wouldn't interfere with getting the story under way. There was a chance, I knew hazily, that I might be out for a while. If I could at least get the piece written and recorded, the producer and film editor could go ahead and cut it without me.

That sounds as if I had come to terms with what might happen to me, but except in the most cerebral, removed way I had not. The borderline panic I had felt in California passed like the sight of a car accident on a highway. A look, a twinge, and onward. It seemed reasonable to react that way. What was the point of worrying about something that probably wouldn't happen? Worry took time and energy. I valued my time and energy. I didn't want to waste it on the fear of something as unlikely as breast cancer. Nine out of ten benign, I reminded myself daily. And there's no cancer in the family. And I'm young. And I'm me.

I did not get the piece written or recorded that day. There was too much film to see, and it was too good a story to rush it through. As I got up to leave, we were looking at an interview with the man who had set up the filming of the AA meeting. It wasn't bad. "Some of these kids feel ugly or awkward or stupid, so they literally hide behind glasses—or cans —of alcohol. . . ."

"That's usable, I guess," I said to the producer. "I'm not sure if we need it, though. What do you think?"

"We can pull it," he said, "and decide later."

I looked at the clock on the wall. Four thirty. My appointment was at five, and the office was on eighty-something street, so it would take about a half hour to get there. Dammit, I thought. "I have to go," I said, getting up.

The film editor pushed the "stop" button. Both men knew that I was going into the hospital for some kind of minor operation. "When will you be in again?" the editor asked.

"Probably at the end of the week," I said. "Do what you can without me, OK?" And I pulled on my coat and ran for the elevator.

Dr. Singermann's office turned out to be in one of the those grand old Fifth Avenue buildings, full of nannies and psychoanalysts. When I got there, Arthur was waiting out in front, under the canopy, smoking. He looked awful. "Don't look so grim," I said, giving him a short squeeze. "It's only a doctor appointment."

Arthur's distress had the odd effect of cheering me up. It was an old perversion. When I was an actress, on stage on an opening night, nothing calmed me more than the sight of an actor who was a wreck. Once, I remember, before making an entrance in the road company opening of *Advise and Consent*, I had a serious case of knee-wobble. That means that, as you walk, your knees give, so that each step is a possible fall. I made it to the onstage bed, when I was supposed to pause and exchange a couple of lines with another actor. As the actor began to speak, I saw that his mouth, his lips—even, remarkably, his forehead—were trembling. It was as if he had a Magic Fingers implant. The poor man, I thought, and then, swift as a miracle cure at Lourdes, my knees were instantly firm. It worked the other way, too. The sight of an actor in repose could, and often did, undo me. It's a matter of emotional role-playing, I suppose, of choosing up sides. If you're easy, I'll take the other part; I'll fidget. If you've got the willies, I'll relax; I'll be gay.

So as I led my shaky husband into Dr. Singermann's dark lobby, I clearly had to be the cheery, tough one. Method actor that I was, I got right into the part. "What an attractive color," I chirped, taking in the deep, not quite forest green of the lobby. "That's the color I wish our draperies were, instead of that awful apple." No response from husband.

I knew why Arthur was upset. He always had a bad reaction to sickness of any kind. I supposed it was because of his mother, now dead, who had been bedridden with crippling arthritis half of her life and most of his. Since his father had left the family when Arthur and his younger brother were small children, and since Arthur was the older, it then became his job to take care of his mother, who was in pain almost all the time. The nights of his childhood, he told me once, were filled with the sound of his mother's moans. Any sign of my ill health—even an upset stomach after too much Chinese food— made him jumpy. Arthur stutters slightly. Whenever I was sick he stuttered more. And he was never especially nice during those times. He would get angry if I wasn't feeling well. Parlor psychology told me he was letting out some of the anger at me that he had felt, but didn't dare admit or express, toward his mother. Still, it made me mad.

He wasn't angry now (and he didn't get angry afterward, either—at least he didn't show it), but he was plenty worried. About me and about himself. After all, here he had married a girl raised to strident good health on her mother's wheat germ, and she turned out (maybe) to be a sickie, like poor old Mom.

But goddammit, I wasn't sick. I felt fine, and the whole business stank of a false alarm.

The office had a Ring and Enter sign under the bell. We rang and entered. I gave my name to the receptionist, and we sat down on two ugly walnut chairs. Ellby's decorator, I thought. I reached for a magazine; at least he had this year's *Newsweek*. And, unlike Ellby's assemblage, there was only one other woman in the waiting room, and she looked dead. I watched her on and off for ten minutes or so, and except for her eyelids no part of her moved. After another fifteen minutes, a nurse called us in.

Dr. Singermann had white hair, glasses, a good jaw, a silk tie, and one oddity: a walleye. His office was small and dark and leathery. He sat behind a desk and I sat in an armchair on one side of the desk, facing him. That left a small chair behind me

36

for Arthur. Without waiting to be asked, I recited the story of my lump—when it was first discovered, what the doctors had said, everything I could think of. Singermann made notes as I spoke and asked me some medical-record kinds of questions: How old are you? Have you ever been pregnant? Is there any cancer in the family? "Absolutely not," was my loud, clear answer to that one. When the questioning was over, I felt that I had done rather well. I gave myself an "A."

Then, almost lazily, the doctor pulled some X rays out of a manila envelope—my mammograms, obviously. He swiveled around in his chair toward the wall, put the shiny black sheets in a viewer, and flicked on a light switch. "Hmmph," he said. "Can't see much on these." He flicked off the switch and swiveled back to face me. "Well, let's have a look," he said, getting up. I followed him into an adjoining examination room. My head buzzed. I felt high. This, I thought, climbing up on the table, is one big charade. I had felt the same silly queasiness so many other times—before a plane landed, or alone in the apartment when something creaked—and always it turned out to be nothing. Nothing at all. And afterward I would always feel like a dumb, jumpy female.

I was on my back and Singermann was palpating my left breast. "Put your arm back." More palpation. Then the other breast. The examination was more thorough than any I had had before, either by

Smith or Ellby. "Sit up, please." More of the same. He moved my arm this way and that, then pushed his fingers into my armpit, as if he were going to pick me up. Then "I'm going to squeeze your nipple now," he said, and did. I knew that if you have breast cancer, the nipple sometimes ejects a fluid. Mine didn't. It didn't even hurt. "You can get dressed now," said Singermann, without a trace of anything dour in his voice. Clearly, I had done as well on the physical as I had on the oral exam.

I flounced back into the chair in his office. Arthur was still in his chair, chain-smoking.

I don't remember exactly how Singermann put it, because, as soon as I got the gist of what he was saying, my head seemed to fill with air and my eyes got hot.

"... definitely something there . . . a mass . . . good chance of malignancy . . . different kinds of mastectomy, as you probably know . . . some women say they want a separate procedure . . . studies show . . . in my own experience . . . but, of course, it's up to you."

He stopped. I realized I was supposed to talk now. It sounded as if I was expected to say whether I wanted just to have my breast cut off, or whether I wanted my breast cut off and some other things too.

Slowly, I turned in my chair and looked at Arthur. Our eyes locked. He told me later he was unable to get the look on my face out of his mind. Not wanting to be rude, I turned back to Singermann. I heard myself speak. "Are you saying that you think I have cancer?" (That word had not been used. I soon learned that cancer is a word doctors almost never use.) "I mean, I know you can't know for sure, but what are the odds—what percentage— what is the likelihood . . . ?"

Dr. Singermann smiled and leaned on his desk. "Everyone wants numbers. It's very hard to say, maybe seventy–thirty, sixty–forty, I don't know."

I heard myself speak again. "Are you saying, do you mean it's sixty or seventy percent *likely*, you mean it's *likely?*"

It was making him uncomfortable. "Look, percentages are just percentages. People want numbers, you give them numbers, but . . . unreliable . . . you don't really know until . . . but . . ." Then he stood up. Then Arthur stood up. Then I stood up. Then I fell down.

I didn't faint, exactly, because I didn't altogether lose consciousness. Nor did I fall far, or get hurt. The office was so small that when Arthur stood up he was only a few inches from me, so that, as I fell, he caught me. There was a small sofa in the room, and I remember being placed on it. It was too short for my legs, so Arthur hung them over the arm of the sofa, like wet towels. "I'll be all right," I said. But the line must have convinced no one because as soon as I said it I began to cry, the bad, loud, gasping kind. I wanted to hold something, so I held my face. I held it hard with both hands, as if it were someone else's. I felt something odd on my cheek. A false eyelash. I put it in the pocket of my dress. (Three months later I found it there, bent and full of lint.)

Singermann had left the room after I fell. I heard his voice now from one of the other rooms outside. "You never know about these things. Her doctor said she could take it. . . . Everybody wants you to be honest . . . and look what happens." I put my hands down, away from my face. ". . . very upset . . . ," I heard Arthur say. "Sixty percent is just a number." That was Singermann.

I sat up. Then I stood up. There was a box of tissues on Singermann's desk. I pulled one out and carefully wiped my face. Arthur came back into the room. "I'm OK," I said, but it came out in a whisper. He put his arm around me, and we walked out of the room slowly, like two old people. The waiting room was empty now, except for the nurse and Singermann. Singermann looked even more uncomfortable than before. I felt embarrassed. "I'm sorry," I said to him, still in a whisper. "I'm all right now.

"Jesus," I said to Arthur as we limped out. "How many times a week do you think he has to do that?" Arthur shook his head and stopped to light another cigarette. The hand that held the match was shaking.

The nice green lobby didn't look nice any more.

The green just looked dark now, like fungus. Outside, the air was strangely warm and soft. There was a breeze. It was all so normal. I started to cry again. The doorman pretended not to notice and hailed a taxi. We got in. Arthur told the driver our address. I put my head back on the seat and closed my eyes. We didn't speak for a while.

"It still may not happen, you know," I rasped. Still no voice.

"That's true," Arthur rasped back. Then we were silent again.

I had sunglasses, thank God, so I could make it from the taxi to the lobby without our doorman's noticing anything. Silence again going up in the elevator. At the door, Arthur fussed with the keys, swore, unlocked both locks, and finally we were inside.

Home. I loved that apartment, our daffy, sweet apartment (over which I had driven two decorators crazy: "It's *not* Versailles, for Chrissake!" the second one had screamed). I looked at my plants in their nice clay pots on the windowsill and started to cry again and stumbled into the bedroom and fell on the bed. Arthur followed me. I should take off the bedspread, I thought. I'll get it dirty, especially if I cry on it. Arthur lay down next to me. He held me with both arms. It felt strange. Arthur didn't do that sort of thing much. It was one of the things I used to complain about. "You never kiss me," I used to say. "You're out of your mind," he'd say.

"I don't mean in bed," I'd say. "That doesn't count. I mean in the kitchen, on the street. You never kiss me on the street." "I do too," he'd say. "You do *not*. Name one time you've ever kissed me on the street." "All right, all right, I'll kiss you on the street." But he didn't.

He was kissing me now, though—on my forehead, on the side of my face where the tears had rolled, and in my hair. I thought of a newspaper interview with Marvella Bayh, the senator's wife who had had a mastectomy, that I had read a few weeks earlier. She talked about her operation bringing her and her husband closer together. It was corny, sort of, but convincing.

Arthur hugged me tighter. Maybe that will happen to us, I thought. Maybe he'll kiss me on the street now.

5

I STARTED CALLING PEOPLE right away. I wanted badly to call my mother, but I didn't call her. Why put her and my father through this, I reasoned the way I had reasoned with myself, if it doesn't happen? After all, I kept repeating shrilly to myself, *it still might not happen!* It was still possible, wasn't it, that I didn't have cancer, that they would send me home from the hospital with a little scar, like Millie's? All right, all right, I had to face the fact that that was no longer probable. But probable didn't mean definite. Probable meant probable. Probable meant it was still possible that I was all right, the way I had always been all right.

I called my best friends, my pseudo-siblings (which is what we only children make of our best friends)—people I love, people who love me back, even when it's not convenient.

I called Leo first. Leo Bloom is an actor. We met seventeen years ago when we were in a dreadful show together on the summer circuit. It was a revival of *Dulcy* by George S. Kaufman and Moss Hart. The star was Dody Goodman. The play never should have been revived and Dody Goodman should have stayed put on the Paar show where she was funny. Anyway, Leo and I found each other that summer. It was never a romance. It was just that—however cloying it may sound—he became the brother I never had, and I became his sister. In the years that followed, when he flunked an audition I would take him to the movies. And when I suddenly decided to leave an artist I was living with in a tenement on East Twenty-first Street, Leo rushed down in a taxi he couldn't afford to help me down five flights of stairs with my suitcases, so that I could get out before the artist (he was sweet, but occasionally violent) came home and, possibly, beat me up. Even when everything was OK, we cooked for each other regularly, and even when we had functioning romances with other people, we would bring each other along. Our respective boyfriends and girl friends thought it was weird, but they got used to it. They had to.

When I told him, Leo lost his voice. (Why are voices always first to go?) He whispered a lot of questions. He wanted every detail—what *exactly* had the doctor said, had I told my parents, etc. When there was no more to ask or say, we hung up.

So now I had made my best friend miserable, too. I felt guilty, but not guilty enough not to make the next call. I called Erica. Erica Abeel, whom I know from Sarah Lawrence, is both my most accomplished and my most fragile friend. She is a professor, a writer, a mother, a beauty, a wit, and a wreck. Erica is almost always on the verge of falling apart. When she heard my news, she nearly did. She, too, began to whisper—and stammer as well. I had never heard her do that. After a few minutes, she tried to say something positive. "M-m-maybe it w-w-won't happen." It didn't work.

Then I called the rest of my college trio of best friends: Joanna Simon, the opera singer, who was my ex-roommate (she wasn't home), and Pat Fischer, who lives in Philadelphia. Pat, like Erica—and like me too, I suppose—is an unlikely blend of sturdy and shaky. When I called her, she was sturdy. "You can absorb this," she said. "If it happens, you can absorb it." She is right, I thought afterward. I can absorb it. I can absorb it. But, oh, God, please don't let there be anything for me to absorb. Please. But praying to God was no good, because long ago I had decided I didn't believe in God, so why should he do anything to help me now?

I lay back on the bed. Calling people had made me feel better. Calls are talking and talking is connecting. And connect was what I wanted to do now. Connect and lean. Arthur was in the kitchen, cooking dinner. I knew I could lean on him, but not a lot. Not as much as I knew I'd need to. Especially if it happened. If.

Arthur Herzog III, author of *The Swarm, Earthsound, The B.S. Factor,* and other peculiar and arresting books, is the most charming man I have ever known. We met at a party two years before we married. He was wearing a pin-striped suit and big glasses and he was imposing and confident and funny and smart and classy, and besides all that he had two irregularities: a small space between his two front teeth and a slight, occasional stutter that tapped my maternal feelings and made me love him right away. He moved into my apartment. When we lived together, he was ever more charming, adorable, smart, sexy, and funny. He was also impossible. He was an artist and everything had to be his way. I decided it was worth it. I wanted to marry him. He did not want to marry me. He had done that a few times before and he said it spoiled everything. Moreover, he thought monogamy was silly. I did what women do: Marry me or lose me, I said. OK, OK, he said, I'll marry you. So we married, one summer in Denmark. We fought a lot. But we laughed more than we fought. He drank a little too much, and he was mean sometimes. But after a while I saw that he talked mean more than he acted mean. Most people talk nicer than they act. Arthur is the opposite. In a way, I loved him for that. I was proud of him for having such lousy public relations. I thought it showed a kind of integrity. Not kissing me in the street or in the kitchen (or buying me flowers or buying me anything much) was part of the same thing. Arthur was thoughtless, the way some men are, and I didn't like that. But Arthur was also just Arthur—not mushy, not smooth, not a butterer-upper. And I liked that. He was on the level. Less than sympathetic, most of the time, but authentic. Besides, my strong hunch was that for all his lack of mush Arthur loved me. And, although the word love has always baffled me when I think about it too hard, I loved him.

Besides, I loved being married. I loved the idea that the person I felt sexy about was, at the same time, my family. I loved those two things coming together. I built a nest on East Fiftieth Street. I felt happy. Sometimes. We did fight a lot. Picky, nasty fights, some of them. I learned to get up the next morning and forget it—until the next one. Some of our fights were about monogamy. He said he didn't want it; I did. He thought I was middle-class; I thought he was disloyal. The fact was that because of the no-rules world we lived in, neither of us was sure what marriage was supposed to be or what we wanted it to be. So we kept testing each other. We learned a thing or two from the testing, but it hurt.

Some of our fights were about what I saw as Arthur's irritability and what he saw as my being irritating. Conversations turned into disagreements turned into fights. We fell into that married people's trap: Our fighting became a habit which neither of us wanted—or knew how—to break. "You never agree with anything I say!" he'd shout. "The only way to talk to you is to agree with everything you say!" I'd shout. He thought I was too critical. I thought he was thoughtless. On and on and on. Nothing happened, either between us or around us, to make things better. So they got worse. Still, we carried on. And in the middle of our uneasy and frenetic carrying-on, I got breast cancer.

6

"HAVE YOU SEEN Gloria Swanson lately?" Eugene asked me. "She looks marvelous. My dear, it's what she eats. Even her grapefruit she has flown in." Eugene was ecstatic. Eugene is my hairdresser and he gets ecstatic a lot. That was one of the reasons I went to him that Saturday morning. The other reason was to get my hair done. If there was about to be a tragic occurrence, I wanted to look nice when it happened.

After the Singermann appointment on Friday, the immediate problem was how to get through the weekend. (I was due at the hospital Sunday afternoon.) Saturday morning, I decided what would get me through the day best: trivia. Besides Eugene, that meant Bloomingdale's. I am not proud of what this says about my character, but I feel really good in Bloomingdale's. I bought an expensive pair of silver earrings. I bought an expensive pair of shoes. I hung around the cosmetics counters and stuck my fingers in pots of lip gloss. Then I went outside. Bright sunshine.

My stomach suddenly flipped. It occurred to me

that the Valium might be wearing off. I went home. Arthur was there, writing. He was working on a book about an earthquake. He came out of the study when he heard me come in. "Are you OK?"

"Not bad," I said. "Just came home for another fix." The Valium was on the bedside table. I took one. "*You* don't look so hot," I told him. He did look awful, worse than I. His imagination, I found out many days later, had gone much further than mine. I was afraid that I might lose a breast. That horror was as far as I could go. Arthur had gone on to the next. He thought—and knew it was reasonable to think—that I might lose my life.

That night we went to the movies with Susan Wood and Joe Haggerty. Susan Wood and Joe Haggerty are the best good-time people I know. Susan, a photographer by trade, is intensely dotty, and Joe, who is Irish, does something in concrete and is adorable when he is sober and more adorable when he is drunk, which he is with some regularity. The movie was a musical with Barbra Streisand. Aside from Barbra Streisand's breasts, it was a perfect movie to see, because it was both silly and absorbing.

Usually I don't drink, but after the movie we went back to our apartment and I drank Scotch and we played backgammon and we giggled and I drank some more and then Joe and Susan left and we were alone again. As soon as the door closed, the giggling stopped and I didn't feel drunk any more. I emptied the glasses in the sink and put them in

50

the dishwasher. Arthur closed the backgammon set. It was very quiet. Suddenly, I felt woozy. I went into the bedroom and lay down on my back and stared at the bump on the ceiling that used to be a light fixture. The wooziness stopped and I got up. I took my clothes off and went into the bathroom where my nightgown was hanging on a hook on the door. I reached for it and stopped. There was a mirror on the door and I looked at myself. I looked at my breasts. They're nice, I thought, they've always been nice. Somewhat small, but small breasts are better for clothes. And they stay up better. I never wore a bra much any more except to go to work. It used to make me self-conscious, at first, that when I was braless my nipples stuck out, but soon I noticed that other women's nipples stuck out sometimes, too, so it stopped bothering me.

When I was young—twelve, thirteen, fourteen—I used to worry that I would be flat-chested. I was smaller than some of the other girls. And those were the fifties, the-bigger-the-better days, when adolescent boys liked you directly in proportion to the size of your bra cup. Perhaps they really didn't. Perhaps it just seemed that way to those of us who were small-breasted. I was dimly aware that the girls with very big breasts suffered, too, in a different way. Imagine being paid attention to just because of two big things hanging off you. When a boy liked one of us little-titted girls, at least we knew it was for us, not our mammary equipment.

My breasts grew a bit bigger in high school and so did I. Then I stopped growing, and so did my breasts. I wasn't sure how to evaluate either my height or my breast size until later. Then, it turned out, they both made the grade. The boys who had been shorter than I grew taller, so I could start standing straight again and stop bending my knees at dances. And the breasts, though not as big as I would have liked, were certainly adequate. Besides, I could make them look bigger with those wired bras that pushed everything together and up, like small offerings.

Then, in the spring of my junior year at college, *Mademoiselle* magazine ended all my worries. A photographer and a small, bony woman who clanged from the many bangle bracelets she wore came up to Sarah Lawrence to find girls to model some of their fall college fashions. I was picked to model a red sweater. I got into it and presented myself to the clanging lady. It was her job to pin and adjust the clothes before the photograph was taken. She looked at my chest and frowned. I looked down at myself, then up at her, not daring to ask what was wrong. She said nothing but went over to a table piled with scarves and jewelry, pulled out a beige silk scarf, and turned back to me. "Lift up," she said, meaning the sweater.

"You mean take it off?" I asked, finding my voice.

"No, just lift up," she said, sounding irritated.

I pulled the sweater up and she began to bind my

breasts with the scarf. After she had made several knots in the scarf, her bracelets making a racket all the while, I decided to speak. "Why. . . ?"

"We're not wearing breasts this year," she snapped. I was thrilled. Imagine being too big-breasted for *Mademoiselle!* After that I knew I was all right.

Now, without taking my eyes off the breast in the mirror, I put my hand over the left one, the one with the lump. I flattened the breast as much as I could, trying to imagine what it would look like if it weren't there. I wondered if they would scoop it out like a melon ball, and whether there'd be a hole. I took my hand away and looked at the breast the way it was. I looked at it as if it were a person I loved whom I would not see again. My throat swelled and my eyes filled up. I pulled my night-gown off the hook and over my head, fumbled in the medicine chest for another Valium, found it, swallowed it, blew my nose, got into bed, and then it was Sunday.

7

THERE IS A LOT of work when you check into a hospital, some of which is busywork, and that's good. Busywork keeps you busy: application forms and blood tests and X rays and cardiograms.

The man who gave me the cardiogram had an accent that I recognized. "You're Haitian, aren't you?"

He looked at me and smiled such an enormous, white-toothed, gorgeous smile that it almost made me feel good. "How you know that?" he said.

"I was there once." Another dazzling show of teeth.

"What you here for?" he asked, after I was wired up.

"Breast cancer." I said, and then I was sorry. He flinched. The smile was gone.

"Oh, you not know for sure," he said. "Maybe you all right."

"That's true," I said. "Maybe I'm all right."

Then an aide escorted me to my room. Arthur came along. The insurance only covered the cost of a semiprivate room, but I had taken a private room anyway. I figured if It Happened, I wouldn't want a roommate. The room was bare and clean, with a window that looked out over the parking lot. I unpacked my suitcase and put everything away, deciding carefully what should go in which place. There was one chair in the room. Arthur sat on it and read the Sunday *New York Times Magazine*. I looked at the bed. That's where I'm supposed to be, I thought. I got undressed and put on my nightgown and got underneath the crisp white sheets. "I feel silly," I said to Arthur. "What am I doing in bed? I'm not even sick." He looked at me, started to say something, didn't, and went back to the paper. But I am sick, I thought. Then I said it again to myself as if I were eight years old and writing it on the blackboard as a punishment for telling a lie. I am sick. I am sick.

Soon it was evening and friends came. Alan Buchsbaum, our architect friend who has a red beard and wears funny sandals, even in the winter, came with Scrabble. And Erica came, shaky and smoking, and smiling oddly and too much. There weren't enough chairs, so Alan and Erica sat on the floor with their knees up. Between Erica and Arthur, the room got as smoky as a singles' bar. (We had closed the door, because you're not supposed to smoke. I had learned my first important hospital lesson. If you're in a private room, you don't have to obey the rules. All you have to do is close the door while you're disobeying them.)

We played Scrabble. I love Scrabble, but after about ten minutes I petered out. "I'm sorry," I said to Alan, who was about to unload a seven-letter word, "I'm just too tired." I did feel tired, which was peculiar because, after taking three Valiums the night before, I had slept nine hours.

It was dark outside the hospital window now. There were only a few cars in the parking lot. Visiting hours were over. Alan and Erica left, not knowing what to say, so not saying much. They closed the door behind them and Arthur stayed, but we couldn't seem to get a conversation going either. It was my fault. I was very distracted. He would start to talk and my mind would wander. I kept thinking the same things over and over: How come if I'm so sick, I don't feel sick. How come this is happening? How come this is happening to *me?* *Is* it happening?

Suddenly, Dr. Singermann walked in. He was on his evening rounds, he said. "How are you?" he asked brightly.

"Fine," I said, just as brightly, anxious to show him it wouldn't be like last time.

He sat down at the foot of the bed and started to talk about the different kinds of mastectomies, the way he had in the office. This time I tried not to let the air in my head get in the way. But he was rattling the whole thing off like an airline stewardess explaining the emergency equipment, and I had to keep stopping him to ask him to repeat things. I felt stupid, especially because I knew so much of what he told me from the reports I had done. But I was selling then, and now I was buying.

Until the nineteen fifties, he said, if you had a malignancy (why don't they *ever* say cancer?) you had a radical mastectomy. That meant removal of the entire breast plus the lymph nodes in the armpit and the pectoral muscles.

"That's the chest muscle, right?" I said.

"Yes," he said not liking the interruption. Then, he went on, there was a simple mastectomy, sometimes called a "total," which was removal of the entire breast but nothing more. A lumpectomy, he said, was the removal of the lump and some surrounding tissue. If there was a malignancy, he said, that was too risky, because there was no way to tell if the malignancy had spread to another place in the breast without removing it. But a "radical," he said, would not be necessary. Studies showed that survival rates between women who had "radical" and "modified radical" surgery were the same. (I remembered reading somewhere that for some time those findings were suppressed by some doctors, who did not want their "radical" patients to know that they needn't have had such disfiguring surgery.)

A "modified radical," Singermann went on without skipping a beat, was the operation he did in most cases, and that was what he had in mind for me. With a modified radical mastectomy, the breast comes off, and some lymph nodes (the ones

57

nearest to the breast, the assumption being that if the cancer had spread to the nodes, it would have spread to the nearest ones), but the pectoral muscles would be left intact. In other words, I translated to myself, my breast would come off, but my chest wouldn't cave in.

Dutifully, he added that, if I wanted, he could do the biopsy alone, and, even if the tumor was malignant, I could have the mastectomy in a separate procedure. I knew some women wanted to wake up after the biopsy, get the verdict, then choose what to do. That struck me as stupid. As far as I or anyone else seemed to know at this point, if there was cancer in the breast, a mastectomy was what you did about it. As to which kind to have, Singermann's suggestion sounded reasonable to me. Anyway, what did I know? I had checked out his reputation and it was good. I had to trust him.

He stopped talking. I felt very, very tired again. I looked at him and decided to say what I had been thinking. "I trust you," I said. "Do what you think is best. But I want to be sure you understand what is important to me. I do not want to die. That's number one. And number two is—I am vain. OK? I am vain. I—I would like not to be very hideous, if—if that's possible." My lower lip started to tremble and I bit it. He said something, I don't remember what, and left.

Arthur took my hand. "You better go now," I said to him. He couldn't seem to talk. He bent down and kissed me on the mouth, a small, dry, quivering kiss, and then he was gone. I was alone now and I felt like Alice, whirring down the rabbit hole. Off with her breast, said the Duchess. I held onto the sides of the bed.

"Hello!" A nurse came in, wheeling a cart. She gave me a paper cup with pills in it.

"What are they?" I asked.

"Something to help you sleep," she said, very bright, very cheery. She wheeled her cart out, and another nurse came in. Blood pressure. Then she left.

Then a nurse's aide came in. She was an elderly black woman, and her movements were slower than the young nurses'. "Good evenin'," she said and smiled. In her arms was a basin and in her hand a razor.

"What's that for?" I asked, horrified.

She smiled again. "I'm goin' to shave your arm," she said in a soft Jamaican accent and sat down next to the bed.

"You mean under my arm."

"Yes," she said, gently raising my left arm, "and the arm too."

"Oh, no," I wailed. "But they're not cutting my arm off! Why do you have to shave my arm?" I tried not to cry, but I felt it coming.

"Now don't you worry, dear," said the woman, gently soaping my arm.

"Won't it grow back all stubby?" I whimpered, looking down as she began.

"Oh, no, missus, the ways I does it, it will look

jus' fine. The ways some people do it, it grow back stubby, but I knows *how!*"

My God, I thought, the woman has pride in her work. Pride in her work! I shut up at once and looked at her and smiled.

It was my last smile for quite a while. . . .

The last thing I remember in my presurgical haze is another woman. I could see her through the bars of my presurgical crib. We were in what must have been a presurgical waiting room. The woman was smiling.

"What are *you* having done?" I slurred.

"Plastic surgery," she slurred back in a voice that sounded young.

"Where?" I asked, trying not to fade out in the middle of the conversation.

"Breasts," she said. "What are you having?"

"Breast," I said.

The evening before, I had asked Dr. Singermann how long the operation would take. He told me that it was scheduled for 9 A.M. and if the tumor was benign I would probably be through and in the recovery room at about 11. Otherwise, he said, lingering on the comma, it would take longer, probably until sometime in the afternoon.

When I awoke in the recovery room, a nurse came into focus. I wasn't altogether conscious, of course, but my brain was working—well enough to figure out that the nurse probably wasn't supposed to tell me anything, but *surely* she wouldn't refuse to answer a little old innocent question like what time is it. You fox, I thought to myself as I asked her the question.

"What time is it?"

"It's three fifteen," she said promptly.

I went back to sleep.

8

I LOOKED DOWN at myself. There was a big bandage wrapped tightly around my chest, a clean white bandage. My left arm was propped up on a white pillow. The sheets were clean and white and pressed. My hospital gown was clean and white and wrinkled. The nurse's hat was stiff and white, and so was her dress. Everything seemed very white, except my mother, my father, and Arthur. That's all I remember of the first day.

The second day I was still drugged, but less so. I didn't feel so hot the second day. I threw up a little, couldn't eat, threw up a little more, and peed almost continuously. The nurse would hoist me up, shove a plastic potty under my bottom, and I'd pee; then she'd take it away until the next time, about twenty minutes later. What a lousy job, I thought, worse than having to make breast sandwiches. But she didn't seem to mind.

The second day I had a dream. It was one I used to have when I was a child. A lot of children have it; it's the you-die-and-everyone-is-sorry dream. There are long and short versions. I had the long version. In the long version, there is a funeral, and everyone comes and cries, of course, and is very, very sorry about all the bad things they did to you. Especially your parents. Even if they didn't do bad things, they are sorry and very, very sad. They talk together about how wonderful you were, lingering over each aspect of your fine character, which takes a long time. Many people are there. You do not know them all. But they are there, anyway, all feeling perfectly rotten.

The back of my hand hurt. There were tubes stuck in it—intravenous. That was what was making me pee so much. There was something else attached to me, too, a plastic sac on my side. I didn't notice it until the nurse said, "Your purse is filling up nicely, dear." I didn't know what the hell she was talking about, but I knew I didn't have a pocketbook in bed, so I looked down and there was this sac with a repulsive yellowish fluid inside. Drainage from the wound, I found out. I decided not to look at it again.

Otherwise, I loved the hospital. For six days I lay there and Got. I got flowers, sweet small arrangements of daisies and baby's breath, big purple peonies, and hulking green plants. I got notes and corny cards and constant (paid-for) attention from private nurses and constant (unpaid-for) attention from everyone else. I got telephone calls and visits and presents. The more I got, the more I wanted and the more I got again. I became an acquisitive pig.

I loved everything I got. I loved the shiny card

with roses on it from the NBC film editors that said in curlicued print:

Thinking of you
and hoping
that you're feeling
much better

and, underneath, fourteen signatures that went up on a slant. I loved the note from Erica: it was so Erica.

Betty dear,
It's a stinking lousy deal, but you're going to be okay. Now it'll all be all right. I think that Pat and I both lived through every minute of this whole thing with you, so if that's any comfort we're still hanging in and so tremendously relieved that you're going to be *completely* [underlined twice] *well* [underlined once]. Just keep remembering that, and don't think about things cosmetic. You're still gorgeous.

I'll call you Tuesday when you're feeling less groggy. I asked Arthur to tell you one very important thing. The day I had my babies, I felt like *Shit* [underlined twice] but the *very next day* [underlined once] I felt *enormously* [underlined once] better, not just gradually better. By this time tomorrow you'll really feel human again and full of spirit and fight. A nurse told me that about the day-after-surgery syndrome, and it helped me so much. We all love you and think of you constantly, Betty dear.   Love Erica

And the note from Marty Linsky, a Boston friend:

> . . . it is an important time to realize that you aren't just flesh and bones—that which makes you different, makes you human, makes you you are those less tangible things—how you feel about yourself, how others feel about you . . .

Nice. And I loved the visits, especially the surprise ones. Especially one from David, a banker from Philadelphia whom I had almost married, but didn't, three years earlier.

David is a bear of a man—tall, black-haired, almost fierce-looking. He is forty-one, seven years younger than Arthur, and about seven times more solemn. When he came to see me, I tried to be amusing. He interrupted me. "You don't have to entertain me," he said, in his gentle, almost rabbinical tone of voice. "I just came to sit here and be with you for a while. You don't have to say anything." He had brought me a doll, a striped terrycloth animal with big ears. He put it next to me on my pillow, and my eyes closed and he sat there for a long time.

It turned out later that that was an important visit.

Other people came, people who were close to me or—like David—had been close to me once, and they brought presents, too. I loved their coming, and I loved the presents. My old roommate, Molly Haskell, came and brought me a pretty address book with Indian drawings, and Susan Wood brought me a leather Mark Cross writing folder that smelled wonderful, and flowers came and kept coming at least twice a day. It was like an ongoing birthday. Or a funeral.

I loved telling the story about how I outfoxed the nurse in the recovery room. I told it over and over, and everyone agreed how clever I was. I told other stories, too, that week. And when I ran out of stories, I told other things. Except when I slept, I talked almost all the time. I talked to everyone who came, the nurses and the nurse's aides, even the ones who didn't speak English. Most of all, I talked to my mother.

I had told Arthur not to tell my mother and father until after it happened. The day I went into the hospital, I called them and said I had an assignment out of town—in Boston. (I thought Boston sounded convincing.) That way, I reasoned, if I didn't have cancer, they wouldn't have to know about any of this. I considered not telling them, even if I did have it, but Arthur had said, "If it happens, you'll need your mother."

At first I couldn't imagine "needing" my mother, but on second thought I could. Besides, she was bound to notice. We shop together. What if we were in Bloomingdale's one day and I wanted to try on a sweater. A dressing room in Bloomingdale's is no place to find out that your only daughter is missing a breast.

So, we decided, if the worst happened, Arthur would tell my parents immediately. Arthur himself got the news directly from Singermann. Right after surgery, Singermann had come up to the lounge where Arthur was waiting and told him. Arthur called my mother first and said he had something important to tell her and my father about me, but he wanted to tell them when they were together. He asked my mother for my father's office telephone number, in order to call him and tell him to join her at home. My mother gave Arthur the number and asked if I was dead. Arthur said no, and called my father. When my father got home, he called Arthur back, and my mother got on the extension phone in the bedroom and Arthur told them. When my mother started to cry, Arthur said that they had to pull themselves together and go right to the hospital because I needed them.

When I woke up in my room after the surgery, my parents were there. My mother smiled and kissed me. She did not cry. Nor did I see her cry the rest of the week. Nor did I ever see her cry about what happened.

My mother told me later that my father cried at home. I don't remember him well those first two days. I think he stayed near the wall most of the time. I guess he didn't know what else to do.

My mother is a big feeler, but she has never been much of a crier. Not in front of me, at least. The only time I can remember her crying was when Arthur and I were living together in my walk-up apartment on 49th Street. It was before we were married, and my mother came up to visit. She was fine until she started to leave, and then, at the doorway, having listened to Arthur make his points about *feeling* married to me even though he wasn't, she stood under the ratty brass fixture we had thought would look so great when we bought it in Tangiers, turned the doorknob, and burst into tears. "If you were a mother," she sobbed, "you would understand!" Exit.

Although tears were rare while I was growing up, lines like that were not, and naturally they drove a wedge between my mother and me. For the longest time, we didn't talk to each other about anything important, because she would wind up saying one of those lines, I would overreact to both the style and the content of the line, she would react to my overreaction, and everybody would wind up with a headache or a stomachache or both. Part of the problem was that in my mother's ferocious striving to give me "everything," she had never considered that giving me "everything" would make me (1) different (from her), and (2) guilty (about what I got). Different and Guilty are not the stuff on which comradeship is built.

Then things got better between us. Getting older helped. Analysis helped. Getting married helped. And now, in a way that I could not have predicted, this crisis helped. Arthur had been right. I needed my mother now and she knew it and I knew it. And my mother is very, very good at being needed.

In the hospital she did exactly what I needed her to do. It wasn't only that she was loving and helpful. Of course she'd be loving and helpful. What impressed me—what dazzled and moved me— was how spirited, how bright-eyed and positive and cheerful she was. Not phony cheerful, either.

"We have to be grateful," she said on the first day —because I was alive. "We have to be very grateful," she said on the second, when the news came that my lymph nodes were clear—which meant that I might stay alive. She, too, talked to everyone else who came in the room. "My daughter's a fighter," she said to one of the Filipino nurses who hardly spoke English. And as the nurse smiled and nodded politely, she said again, "My daughter's a fighter."

My mother said most things twice like that. But that was OK. I didn't mind. In fact, I liked it. The repetitions underlined her spunk. And her spunk was magnificent. She bustled about a lot, those days in the hospital. She ran the shop. She brought me things when a nurse wasn't around, and sometimes she brought them when the nurse was around. She answered the phone and handled the calls I didn't want to take with the aplomb of a social secretary. If a flower from one of the many bouquets I got showed a sign of wilting, if a leaf turned even vaguely yellow, she plucked it.

She listened to me. And I listened to her. We

talked about the past. Sometimes we got mushy. One late afternoon when I was coming off Demerol I looked at my mother, rearranging the flowers for the fourth time that day. She was humming. Hey, Mother, I thought, I love you. Then I decided to say it. "Hey, Mother, I love you and I'm glad you're here and I think you're being terrific."

"Don't be silly," she said briskly, as she clipped off some leaves with a pair of shears she had brought from home. "What are mothers for?"

I got many congratulations for being so brave and cheerful. I liked that, so I got more brave and more cheerful. And the more brave and cheerful I was, the more everyone seemed to love me, so I kept it up. I became positively euphoric.

It pleased me, in a way, to hear about others who were not as heroic as I. I lapped up stories one of the nurses would tell me: about a woman who, for two entire days—forty-eight hours after her mastectomy—kept her eyes shut; about another woman, a doctor's wife, who went home after her operation and stayed there without going out once for six months. I pretended to feel sorry for those other women and for a few seconds I suppose I did, but these tales carried with them built-in congratulations for me for not being like the person in the story, and my chief reaction when I heard about their inability to cope was shameless, narcissistic, vain, self-congratulatory, competitive pleasure.

I got something else in the hospital I liked, too:

pity. Not that I got nearly as much pity as I did congratulations. Nor did I get nearly as much pity as I would have liked. People think that people who have awful things happen to them don't want pity and, further, that pity is not good for people. They are wrong. That disreputable myth was started, I suspect, by some relative of a disaster victim who didn't want to bother. Pity is delicious. I was crazy about the pity I got. It was the best kind, too. I did not get, nor did I want, the drooling, mewing kind. I preferred something more restrained but deep-felt. Quality pity.

Aside from the pleasure I got from pity itself, it also served as a splendid lead-in for my brave act. All I needed to hear was a slightly choked, "Betty, my God, I just heard, I can't tell you how sorry . . ." and there was a perfect cue for "I'm feeling terrific, absolutely terrific, being spoiled to death—oops, guess that's not the *best* way to put it—heh, heh . . ." and so on.

My favorite telephone call of that kind came from a woman friend who said, "I hear you're coping, and I don't know how. I think I'd just plain die."

"No, you wouldn't," said I, revving up for another favorite role, the Strong One. "If you have a choice, one thing you absolutely don't do is die." Then I would segue nicely into my Pollyanna routine.

Remember that creep, Pollyanna, the Glad Girl? During the week of April 7, 1975, in Beth Israel

Hospital on the surgical ward in Room 343, the spirit of Pollyanna was born anew within the newly mangled frame of Betty Rollin. Most of the time I was too busy in the hospital even to think about anything so downbeat as the fact that I was now missing a breast. But when I did think or talk about it, the Glad Girl kept shining through: I'm glad I only lost one breast instead of two; I'm glad I was sort of flat-chested to start with, so it won't look all *that* different; I'm glad it doesn't hurt much (no doubt about it, a good dose of pain and Pollyanna would have closed out of town); I'm glad it won't show when I'm dressed, say the way an arm or a leg or a nose would; and, oh, yes, I'm glad I'm not dead and—well, who needs a breast, anyway, you can't *do* anything with a breast, you can't type with it or walk on it or play "Melancholy Baby" with it? And besides all that, a breast is something you have two of, so if it serves a purpose (I did remember vaguely that it figured in sex) there's still the other one.

In the hospital I remember having almost no thoughts and only one conversation with Arthur about sex. "Do you still love me now that I only have one?" I asked, coy as all get out.

"Of course, baby," he said and gave me a kiss. I believed him, because he sounded convincing and because what he said was nice. I wanted to (and did) believe and hear everything that was nice. If, conversely, it wasn't nice, I didn't believe it, didn't hear it, and I certainly didn't think about it. Not yet.

Speaking of sex and love and such, throughout the haze of the drugs and the flowers and the nurses and the bandages and the tubes, something else, both very odd and very exciting, was going on: David kept coming back to see me, and he kept staying longer and longer. He'd wait for Arthur not to be there, and then he would come and stay as long as he could before Arthur came back.

On the third day, Arthur noticed. "I don't like that guy hanging around," he said. "What's he doing here, anyway?"

"I don't know," I said. But I did know, because he told me. He said he was in love with me. That was not a big surprise. He had told me that three years ago, just before I married Arthur, and he told me after I had married Arthur, too, but not right away. Knowing how he felt about me, I had avoided him during most of my marriage. But during the past few months, as things got more difficult and more confusing with Arthur, I had avoided him less.

And now, here he was in the hospital, and I was avoiding him not at all. In the past, I had never known quite what to make of David or his feelings for me. He had never married; nor had he ever lived with anyone, except for a very short time; and never, he said, had he ever been in love with anyone

—except me. "Nonsense," I used to say. "It's just that I'm unavailable." But he would shake his head and say, "Try me."

I wasn't about to. But after a fight with Arthur, I'd catch myself daydreaming about it. Then I'd stop. Guilt—and wariness—made me stop. But my doubts about David's feelings for me decreased as my need for them increased. And now, in the hospital, I didn't seem to have any doubts at all. Nor was I guilty. How could I feel guilty about *anything* I did after what had been done to me?

Later, because I wanted badly to explain it to myself, I tried to explain it to Erica. "If what happened to me had happened to you, and the only white horse that had ever been allowed inside Beth Israel Hospital arrived in your room with a prince on it, would you throw him out, just because you happened to be married to someone else?" Guess not, said my pal Erica. Guess not is right. I wasn't throwing anybody or anything out. Especially a man who said he loved me. Especially now.

I wanted to look pretty in the hospital, not only for my flirtation, but for myself. I spent a lot of time looking at my face in the mirror and doing things to it. I rouged my cheeks and plucked out a new line on my eyebrows. At night I put pink rollers in my hair. When my mother overdid it as usual and brought me four new nightgowns instead of the two I had asked for, I did not scold her, as I nor-

mally would, but told her I would like to have a
bed jacket, too. My usual preference in nightgowns is plain and sliplike. But now I liked the
sweet ones my mother brought, with small rosebuds
and lace collars. That was because I wanted to look
pretty in a particular way: fragile. Fragility, I
thought, would complement my stoicism.

Although I lay in bed looking like Ophelia,
what came out of my mouth sounded increasingly
like Ernest Borgnine. An unsuspecting visitor
would tiptoe in and, as likely as not, hear "Step
right up, folks, and see the titless wonder!"

While I was in the hospital I almost never used
the word "breast," it was tit this and tit that. Rough-
tough talk was not only part of my increasingly
agile defense, it was also another good crowd-
pleaser. Whatta girl, I'd hear them think. Whatta
sensa humor. What guts.

I talked tough to Singermann too. He took it in
stride. "How are you today?" he asked on his
rounds one morning, after I had just thrown up my
Cream of Wheat.

"Shitty," I said. Then, thinking better of it, I
said, "Lousy."

"I know what shitty means," he said huffily.
From then on, we almost never had a conversation
that was not laced with four-letter words.

Singermann also congratulated me for having
such a good-looking wound and for healing so
nicely. (I suppose he was really congratulating him-

self, but I didn't read it that way at the time.) As far as having an attractive wound, I had to take his word for it, because I wasn't about to look. Most of the time, I *couldn't* look because I was bandaged. When he changed the bandage I could have looked, but I didn't. I was not even tempted. I'd sit on the edge of my bed and he'd unwrap me and we'd yammer away in our usual language (tit, shit, fuck, et al.) and I would pick a dirt spot on the window and, as more and more of the wrapping came off, I'd stare harder and harder at the spot. I knew what I was doing. I knew that one look might blow my whole act, and I wasn't going to do that. My act was all I had.

9

THE NURSES, it seemed, talked a lot or almost not at all. Moreover, the amount of rhetoric seemed to break down along racial lines. The Filipinos talked the least. I had two Filipino nurses, both young and both very pretty. First I thought they didn't speak because of English language problems. But it soon became apparent that they did, indeed, understand English, and, when it was necessary, they did speak. They simply chose not to speak when it was not necessary. I could tell by the way they smiled and did things (perfectly, with astonishing grace) that their silence was not unfriendly or hostile. Rather it seemed to come from a kind of sweet humility. They seemed to think they *shouldn't* talk unless they had to. Imagine!

The night nurses were mostly black, elderly women, and they didn't talk much either. Nor were they unfriendly. As with the Filipinos, silence just seemed to be their style. Besides, it was night.

The elderly white day nurses made up for the others. Of these, the chattiest by far was a four-foot-nine Italian whose name plate said something very like Saltimbocca, which is a good veal dish. Saltimbocca told me all about herself. She told me, with a good deal of pride, that she had been at Beth Israel for twenty-seven years; that she lived alone; that she loved television, and that she especially loved Lawrence Welk. (It was Saltimbocca who told me about the mastectomy patient who wouldn't open her eyes. She had other grim tales in her repertoire, which she loved to tell and which I loved to hear.)

Saltimbocca was my first nurse after the surgery and she was wonderful. As drugged as I was at first, I had an immediate sense of her. She was like my mother—warm, upbeat, efficient, and bustling. Her little mouth was set and her little arms were strong. She also had what she called a special "little trick" to make her post-ops feel better. She was proud of her trick, as well she should have been. After surgery—whatever kind—your mouth is very dry, painfully, agonizingly dry, but you are not supposed to have water because you might throw it up. So most patients just lie there, with cracked lips and a tongue that feels as if it's licked all the carpets in Persia, begging for water and not getting it. Saltimbocca didn't give me water, but her "little trick" was to wet my mouth with Q-tips soaked in glycerine. The relief was exquisite.

She didn't talk all that much at first, or maybe I was too drugged to notice, but after a day or two she was a hurricane of chitchat. Between her and my mother—and then me—the room began to sound like the birdhouse in the Bronx zoo.

There was another white day nurse who talked almost as much as Saltimbocca, but who was not in the least lovable. She was sort of a cross between Molly Goldberg and Mussolini. "Today," she'd thunder, putting her face near mine and grabbing the hand on my good arm, "I want you to *eat!*" Or, "Today, I want you to *walk!*" It was she who weaned me too early from the potty, and it was onto her small frame (she was another under-five-foot ninety-pounder) I fell, when I passed out on my way to the toilet. The last thing I remember before landing was her screaming "Rose! Rose!" Rose turned out to be the name of the nurse next door, but it caused me to hallucinate briefly about being in a garden. When I came to, I was back in bed with smelling salts under my nose. That surprised me, because I thought smelling salts were only used in plays.

I don't know if I ever actually peed. Or where.

It was back to the potty the rest of that day, but corridor perambulation began the next. I got all dressed up for my first stroll. I had a white dotted-swiss robe that I had bought on sale in Henri Bendel's the year before. It had been too sweet and too white for any previous occasion in my life. Given my wish to look like Sleeping Beauty, however, it was (I felt) perfect for my hallway debut. I checked myself out in the mirror over the washbasin. Then, with my little mother on one side and little Mussolini on the other, I loomed into the hallway.

Beth Israel is no Doctor's Hospital or Lenox

Hill. The corridors do not teem with Beautiful People. There were, as far as I could see to the waiting room, wheezing, bent, unshaven elderly men, in faded pajamas, noiseless except for the shuffling sound of their worn black plastic slippers.

On one of my walks, Saltimbocca nudged me and cocked her head at a woman coming my way. "That's another one," she hissed in my ear. "She had what you had."

"No kidding?" I said, delighted. I stared at the woman as she came nearer. She had dark hair and a beak nose. She wobbled slightly on the arm of a tall young man who looked like a son. Her hair was a mess and she did not look agreeable. But never mind; to me, she was another Porsche owner in the next lane. I gave her one of my manic smiles. "How are *you?*" I leered. She stared at me for a moment as if I were mad, nodded, tried to smile, didn't make it, mumbled "Fine," and shuffled on. That was my last try at making friends in Beth Israel. Except for the jolly rabbi.

My married name, stuck on the door outside my room, was unmistakably Jewish; Arthur, actually, is half Jewish, and the half that's Jewish is the snooty German kind that does not like to make much of it. Nevertheless, the name is Herzog and for that reason, I suppose, the rabbi came to call. When he announced who he was, I was stunned. I hadn't seen a rabbi up close in years and said so. He might have been offended, but he wasn't. He just smiled, baring a hideous set of mostly pointed, yellow teeth, and said, "Is that so!"

Arthur was in the room at the time and looked up, horrified. I'm sure he thought I was up for last rites. I tried to think of something friendly to say. "Well," I began, "we're one and a half Jewish!"

"Is that so?" he said again, and backed out.

I hoped he would come again, but he didn't. His visit made me think about being Jewish. I don't know what it means, never really have, and at various times in my life, in varying degrees, that has bothered me. I stopped believing in God at about the same time I stopped believing in Pinocchio, when I was about eight. It upset my mother because her father was an Orthodox rabbi. My mother blamed herself for not emphasizing religion enough and for not keeping a kosher house. (She couldn't do that, she said, because the housekeeper was a German Catholic and didn't know how. Even at the time, that struck me as a limp excuse.) Later I came to think that one reason I never had much truck with religion was that my mother, in spite of her carryings-on, didn't either. Mother was too hard-headed for that sort of thing, and so was her hard-headed daughter. My father was both more religious and more tribal. I expect that was owing to his experiences in Russian pogroms. When I was little he used to tell me stories about how he and his brothers and sisters hid under beds when the Cossacks came to the houses of the Jews. The

Cossacks would thrust their swords into the mattresses; my father told me that once, when he was under the bed, the tip of the sword came through right next to his head. A rich relative got the family out, but such experiences stick.

For my father, it was always the Jews and the "others." Besides, he liked to sing, and at Jewish holidays he got to sing in the temple.

Not believing in God did not help me solve the Jewish-identity question. That is, one was an atheist—well, an agnostic (who knows for sure?)—but still one was Jewish, no? Yes? When I was in high school I decided that I wouldn't be Jewish because I didn't want to be like some of my friends' mothers who had mink stoles. And for a long while I didn't get attracted to any boys or men who were Jewish. For about ten years, everybody I fell for had a first name like Blair or Kurt, last name to match, bomber-pilot jaws, and, more often than not, infantry minds. (It was the female version of the frequent and noncoincidental preference on the part of Jewish males for German or Swedish airlines stewardesses, even when they're not pretty.) I got over that, but it didn't solve the problem or answer the question. I now wanted to be Jewish—I suppose because the smartest and the nicest people I knew seemed, mostly, to be Jewish—but I still didn't know what it meant. (Still don't.) I thought about all this in the hospital because I knew that disasters often made people religious.

After all, had I not sort of prayed the weekend before?

One hears about people who "turn to God" when the jig is up. Notwithstanding my one prayer, that didn't seem to be happening to me. But then my jig wasn't up, and it still had not occurred to me that it might have been, or that it might yet be.

I kept needing to talk. My mother wasn't there all the time any more, Saltimbocca had a new charge, and Arthur only came in the evening. Besides, he was still too much of a wreck to talk much, and he was never a great listener.

At first I didn't telephone people, because I couldn't decide whom or whether to tell. But when a constant audience was no longer present in the room, there was only one thing to do: call the audience up. A beige princess phone was within easy reach on the night table. Six or eight times a day, I'd sit up, dial a number, lie back on the pillow and say, "Hi! Guess where I am and what happened to me!"

Soon people began calling me back. The calls exhausted me, but I liked getting them. I needed them. Talking became a kind of drug. The other kinds of drugs kept me from feeling physical pain, and talking kept me from the other kind of pain. As long as my mouth was moving, I didn't have to think. Or feel.

Some incoming calls took me by surprise. One

came late on Saturday night. Arthur had just left, and I was staring at the ceiling, gathering energy to get to the sink to brush my teeth, and the phone rang. "Hello," I said.

"How the hell is anyone supposed to find you if you're registered under your married name?" barked a male voice.

"Who is this?" I asked.

"Wald," barked the voice.

"Walt who?" I said.

"Richard C. Wald," came another bark. Richard C. Wald is the president of NBC News.

"How come you're calling me up?" I said.

"I'm at home and I was just thinking about you."

"Gee, that's really nice," I said, meaning it. And although the conversation was all wisecracks and tough talk, afterward I was very touched by it. Wald is very steely. He has to be. "You probably won't make it," he said when I first came to NBC from *Look*. But during the next two years, he did everything to help me prove him wrong.

"Remember when you were a skinny kid who talked through her nose?" he said to me in his office one day, after I had been made a network correspondent. "Yop," I said. "I *still* talk through my nose sometimes." And he gave me a good hard smile that I knew was not all steel.

What touched me about his telephone call, as I told him a month later when I ran into him in the hallway, was that he didn't have to make it. He could have done an appropriate Boss number and sent flowers and written a nice note. He didn't have to call me on the telephone on a Saturday night. "Think of the risk," I told him. "When something like that has happened, you never know how the person is going to be when you call. Suppose I was in some sort of *state*. Suppose I was crying?"

"I'd have told you to stop," he said, and sprinted down the hallway.

So he knew. That meant other people at NBC knew. I didn't mind. More people knowing meant more attention. But it also meant more people getting upset, like Erica, and that bothered me. Erica told me later why, in part, she was so upset. "I figured if it could happen to you, it could happen to me," she said. "I never stopped feeling myself up those first few days you were in the hospital."

A lot of women reacted that way—fearful about themselves. They put it differently but I could see it in their faces—or hear it as their voices cracked. I didn't blame them, and sometimes I encouraged them to be afraid. "I'm not trying to scare you," I'd say, gearing up for my mammogram commercial, "but you should be *sure* to get mammograms at least once a year. And you should examine yourself once a month after your period." Then I'd stop, when I saw them get pale.

I got another kind of reaction from women: I'm sorry for you, but thank God it's not me. No one said that, of course, but I saw them think it. At first, it made me angry. But it made me less angry when I realized I had felt the same way about the bad turns in other people's lives. Now it was my turn to be the object of those ignoble feelings.

I had known what it is to be envied by women. It was odd, now, to face women and hear them think: I'm glad I'm not you.

Not that I felt like a victim. While I was in the hospital, outside of some early physical pain and lingering discomfort, I didn't feel much of anything. I knew what had happened to me, but only between the ears. I didn't know emotionally. Moreover, I didn't know that I didn't know. I thought what everyone else thought, that the reason I wasn't upset was that I was so gutsy and terrific. I had no cause to challenge that explanation. Besides, I liked thinking that about myself.

My thinking was definitely peculiar. I thought a lot, but I couldn't seem to fasten my mind directly on what had happened. Nothing stuck.

Even when there was good news, I heard it but I didn't quite get it. When, for example, the extremely good and crucial bulletin came, forty-eight hours after surgery, that my lymph nodes were clear (which meant that the cancer had not spread, thereby tripling my chances of survival), I hardly reacted.

This numbness surely had something to do with drugs. (I was on Demerol first, then back to Valium.) But drugs or no drugs, numb was clearly what I wanted to be: numb and helpless. I had a sense of having lost control, but it was not an unpleasant sense. Something bad had happened to me. Now it was over. There was nothing I could do about it. There was nothing I could do about it before it happened, either, but before, I was afraid. And to be afraid is in a way to be hopeful, because to be afraid means that you haven't given up. You know it doesn't help, but you keep thrashing. The monster has you pinned to the wall, but you're not ready to say, "Oh, hell, eat me."

Now I was in the monster's stomach. And it wasn't so bad. He had a nice little bed there for me, with sides, like a crib, and plenty to eat. It was warm, and I was sleepy. "Betty was such a happy baby," my mother used to say. In the monster's stomach I was happy and good. I was also cute and I smiled and I cooed and obeyed and everyone loved me. And I wasn't afraid any more, because the thing I was afraid of had happened. Now I could just lie there and let the grown-ups worry.

I never felt the classic "Why me?"—not even during the bad days that were to follow, not even when I was feeling the sorriest for myself. Odd as it sounds, I think that it had something to do with the Vietnamese war, which happened to be ending while I was in the hospital, and like everyone else I watched it on television. I watched those wretched scenes of people clawing to get out, and, also like everyone else, I had seen all the other wretched scenes of that war, for weeks, months, years, before it was finally over. During all of that time, I thought, as everyone thought, "Why them?" Why anyone, but mostly, "Why them?" Why should those people suffer so much for so long? I marveled at the pure unluckiness of being born a Vietnamese in the twentieth century.

I had had "Why them?" feelings before, about other people. I had them every time I saw or heard or read about anyone suffering just because they happened to be at the wrong place at the wrong time with the wrong color skin or the wrong name. And if you feel, "Why them?" it is logical to feel, "Why not me?" There isn't a Jew alive who happened *not* to be in Hitler's Germany who hasn't thought "Why not me?" at least once. One is grateful, of course, but the question persists: Why was I, why am I, so fortunate? Why does lightning always strike where I am not?

So if you are an American, a sheltered, over-privileged, magnificently fortunate American, and one day you get hit; you suffer, you cry, you moan, and you groan; you think, "Why now, why so soon?"—but you can't rightfully think, "Why me?" I felt that losing a breast was lousy, but I never felt that losing a breast was unfair. Not really.

10

APRIL 14. Spring. The air was so warm and sweet, it made me queasy. I had on the same pea jacket I had worn when I came to the hospital the Sunday before. (Was it only a week?) It felt heavy. My shoes felt heavy, too, and tight. All my clothes felt funny. My father was double-parked in front of the hospital. His head was out the window and he looked anxious. I couldn't tell if he was anxious about me or about being double-parked. My mother and Arthur helped me into the back seat. I felt like an old lady. My mother got in the front seat and my father started the car and we moved up Third Avenue. Nobody talked. I looked out the car window, the way I usually do on a trip in the taxi from the airport. I looked at the people. They looked busy. It made me tired just to watch them. I sat back. Then we went over a bump and it hurt, so I sat forward the rest of the way.

The apartment was stuffy, as if we had both been gone for a long time. I pushed open a window. "Don't do that!" said my father, and Arthur and my mother ran over as if I were about to jump out. "There's nothing wrong with my *right* arm," I said, sounding more irritated than I meant to, and then got busy with the flowers. We had brought back all the plants and a few flower bouquets. Some of them were drooping. I began to pull those out and combine the healthy ones that were left.

"Do you have to do that now?" said Arthur.

"Yes," I said.

"How about some nice soup?" said my mother.

"It's only eleven o'clock!" I snapped, pulling out a good flower by mistake.

"Why don't you go to bed?" said Arthur.

"Because I just got out of bed!" I tried to put the good flower back in the bouquet and the stem broke. "Oh, shit," I said. Suddenly, I felt very tired. "I think I *will* go to bed."

"Good," said my mother too enthusiastically. "You don't want to wear yourself out the first day."

The bed felt so wide and soft. I loved that bed, and all the more for having bought it on the phone. Arthur and I were about to go to Europe and get married and when we came back we were supposed to move into this apartment, and just before we left I realized that we didn't have a bed. "Well, go get one," said Arthur. "There's no time!" I wailed. Then I remembered Macy's. My mother always swore by Macy's furniture department. I called them. A man answered. "I am desperate," I said. "I'm getting married and I don't have a bed and I don't have time to come in and pick one." "What kind of bed do you want?" "The best and the biggest," I said. "Leave it to me," he said.

And when we got home from Europe, it was there. And it *was* the best and the biggest. "If we get divorced," I used to say, "can I keep the bed?" "Nope," said Arthur.

I fell asleep. When I woke up, my parents were gone. Arthur came in and sat on the edge of the bed and looked at me. I felt strange. I could tell that he did, too. We kept not having anything to say to each other.

Erica came over for dinner. After she left, Arthur and I had a fight. I don't remember what about.

We made love that night anyway. I wasn't sure if it would be technically manageable, with me in a harness, hurting and sore in front, numb under the arm. But we accomplished it. He needed it, I endured it. There was one part of it I couldn't endure: I couldn't endure his touching my one breast. Poor Arthur, it wasn't his fault. He touched me to be nice, I know, or maybe he even wanted to. But when he cupped his hand and gently held me there, I screamed. I couldn't help it. Feeling his hand on that breast reminded me too much of the other one, the dead twin. Afterward, I dragged myself into the bathroom, took a Valium, and slept through the night.

The next morning I went under, down to the bottom. It was a fast drop. It happened after breakfast. When I woke up, I went into the kitchen. I made coffee and boiled an egg. I ate the egg and drank the coffee. Maybe it was the eerie normalcy of having breakfast, of hearing the typewriter in the next room, or maybe it was that I was alone— no nurses fussing about, no hospital noises, no congratulations, no more salutations for bravery. I was home now, washing out my own coffee cup. I was supposed to be all right. But I wasn't all right. I walked into the living room, sat down in the middle of the long sofa, and started to think.

I started at the beginning and thought about everything that had happened. I thought about the early appointments with Smith, the mammograms, and the first Singermann appointment. I tried to remember what he had told me then, I thought about the report on my lymph nodes, and I went over it all again. I tried to figure out why it happened, and when that didn't work I tried to figure out what was going to happen. The more I thought, the more I realized I didn't know. I didn't know where I was. I knew I was on my sofa, I knew I was back in my life, but I still didn't know where I was.

I went back into the bedroom, sat on the edge of the bed, and dialed Singermann's number. He got on the phone. I wanted to be brief, efficient. Doctors are busy people. "I have to ask you a question," I said. "You've probably already told me the answer, but I don't seem to know it, and—I'd really like to."

"What's the question?" he said.

"I guess I want to know if—if I'm all right now.

I know the lymph nodes were clear and that means chances of recovery are good. But how good? I mean—what are the chances that I won't die?" (I didn't want to sound dramatic, but what other word was there?)

"Well, they're good," Singermann said. "They're very good."

"How good?"

He knew what I wanted. "Eighty to ninety percent," he said.

"Thank you, Dr. Singermann," I said, and we hung up. I was still on the edge of the bed.

I subtracted eighty from one hundred. Twenty. There was a twenty percent chance that I would die. I knew I was supposed to be happy and grateful for the eighty to ninety percent, the way I was in the hospital. But I didn't feel happy and grateful. I had misunderstood what everything meant. I had thought clear lymph nodes meant I was safe, like other people. I thought I was a ninety-six percenter, like everyone else. You can still get killed in a car accident or in a natural disaster, but if you're young and healthy, there is about a ninety-six-percent chance that you will live out your life.

I'm not one of those people any more, I thought. I'm not healthy. I subtracted again. I had gone from a four-percent death chance to a twenty-percent death chance. Five times more chance of dying. My hands were cold. I put them on my neck, which was warm.

Then I picked up the phone again. I called Dr.

Smith. He got on right away. "I'm sorry to . . ." I decided to quit apologizing. "Look, do you have a minute?"

"Yes," he said.

"Well, I just talked to Dr. Singermann, and he said something that disturbed me quite a bit. He said that there's a twenty percent chance that I'll die, and—I mean that's not news and I know I'm supposed to be grateful, but I just wasn't really aware of it before, and I know it's too late and it doesn't matter any more, but would my chances have been better if that lump was taken out when you—we—first found it? I mean, *why wasn't that lump taken out a year ago?*" I tried very hard not to let my voice go up any more. "It was cancer then, wasn't it? Wasn't it? *How come I sat around for a year with cancer?*"

A nurse came in on the line: "Dr. Frank is calling."

"Tell him I'll call him back," snapped Dr. Smith. "Look, Betty," he said in a very low voice, "we're dealing with medicine that is very primitive. You might have had it for two years. You might have had it for two months. We don't know whether that lump was cancer when you first had it. We don't know when you first had it. . . ."

I stopped listening. I was getting that airy feeling in my head again, the one I had had in Singermann's office when he first told me. I hung up. Two thoughts, two sentences, were now inside of me and expanding like a balloon. My head felt as if it were about to split open. One sentence was: If the lump was cancer a year ago, it should have come out then. The other was: If the lump was not cancer a year ago, it should have come out then.

My hands were still cold, but my face was hot. I could hear the sound of the typewriter in the next room. Then, for the first time since the operation, I started to cry.

11

THERE WAS A RULE in our house, a do-not-bother-Daddy-when-he's-working rule. I decided to break it. Arthur looked up when I came in, obviously startled, and moved the lever on the electric typewriter to "off." The house was suddenly still. He waited for me to say something but I couldn't speak right away.

"Arthur," I finally said in a voice smaller than the one I usually use, "It's silly, but I'm all of a sudden worried about dying and will you go out with me for a walk?"

Arthur got up and put his arms around me. "Sure," he said.

I went back to the bedroom and pulled on a pair of pants and a sweater. Getting a sweater on wasn't easy. I was still bandaged, and even though my arm was free I couldn't raise it. There is nothing intrinsically awful about not being able to raise your arm, but as I squirmed to get the sweater on and couldn't, it upset me so much I started to cry again, and then it was even harder to get it on.

After struggling for another full minute, I threw

the sweater on the floor and put on a shirt. But a shirt would be cold. I was always cold now. I was anemic. That was because of the blood lost during surgery. Hospitals don't give transfusions any more the way they used to, because so many people wind up with hepatitis. They give you small green iron pills instead. They work, but they take longer. It would be at least two months, I was told, before my red blood count would be what it was. Meanwhile, you are weak—and cold.

I found a cardigan sweater and put that on. And a bulky jacket that hid my lopsided chest. And sunglasses to cry behind. Which I did (was it the fourth time in an hour?) as soon as we hit the street. Streets are so normal. I think that's why they kept bothering me. I couldn't bear it, after what had happened to me, that everything outside had remained exactly the same: the same small row of shops at the end of the block, the same plants from the plant store spilling over the sidewalk, the Italian vegetable and fruit market with the same overpriced raspberries, the same swirl of people, moving down and up the street with the same unnerving briskness. And there, too, was the grotesquely pretty, midday sunshine.

My lips were dry. I felt as if I were already dead, come back like a ghost, or like the character in *Our Town,* to the street where I once lived.

Through the dark blur of tears and sunglasses I could see on the opposite corner a small, wiry homosexual with a small, wiry dog, the kind you're afraid of stepping on. As we waited for the light to change, I stared at the dog. The reason I stared at the dog was that I felt like the dog. I felt that fragile. I felt as if someone might step on me. When we got to the other side of the street, Forty-ninth and Second Avenue, near the old apartment where I had lived, alone and then with Arthur, the apartment where my mother had cried that day, I started to cry again.

Poor Arthur. Not only had I severed his working day, but he had to walk the streets with a sniveling ghost. As we headed toward the East River, I looked at him. He was gray in the face himself. He looked old.

I couldn't stop crying. And I couldn't get my mind off the numbers—*the* number: eighty. Eighty percent. I began babbling about the number, then about Smith and Ellby. We were walking faster now. "I can accept what's happened," I said hoarsely to Arthur, but really to myself, "but I can't accept that they made a mistake. I can't accept that I live in New York and that I did a story on breast cancer and that I am surrounded with the best, the best doctors, the cream of the medical profession, and that I walked around for a year with a lump in my breast that was cancer. Don't you see? That's what I can't accept." Arthur nodded. He started to say something, then thought better of it. He was right. I didn't want to listen. I wanted to talk, to retch, to vomit words, and that's what I was doing, all over New York's smart East Side, down Forty-ninth Street toward First Avenue, across the street past the United Nations, past the Indians looking up at the tall buildings, and past the Japanese and the Lebanese and past the budding trees and the benches and the guards.

"Maybe we better head home now," said Arthur carefully.

"Yes," I said, knowing how much he wanted me to shut up, and we said nothing on the way back.

How much more of this can he take? I wondered. I didn't want to do this to him, but I had to do it to someone and I didn't have anyone else to do it to. Poor Arthur. Poor Arthur. Poor Betty. How did I get to be a ghost?

When we were back inside the apartment, I pulled off my clothes and threw them on a chair and put on a robe and went back to the phone.

"What are you doing?" said Arthur.

"Calling Larry. I've got to talk to someone who knows something." Larry is Lawrence Cohn, medical doctor, friend, nice guy. He let us know somewhere along the line that he was there, that he would come if I whistled. I whistled. And later that afternoon, he came. By then I wasn't crying any more, but I had the shakes. Leg and stomach shakes.

Arthur asked Larry if he wanted a drink. He had a Coke and sat down on the sofa. I sat next to him.

"Larry"—I tried to sound normal—"I need to talk about numbers," I said, and told him about the eighty percent.

His voice was low, calm, kind. It was also the voice doctors use when they talk to crazy people. "I think the figure for early detection cases is eighty-five percent," he said quietly.

"Larry," I shouted without meaning to, "I had a lump for a year! I'm no early detection case. I'm—"

He interrupted me without raising his voice. "Technically, you *are* an early detection case because the malignancy"—he didn't say cancer either —"didn't spread to the nodes. Early detection means that the malignancy is caught before it spreads, even though it was not, literally, caught early. There is also the possibility," he went on, "that the lump was not malignant at first, so it is possible that your case was more 'early detection' than you think."

"But Larry," I said, trying to fit the pieces together—it was as if I had woken up from a week-long sleep—"if the lump wasn't malignant, then taking it out might have meant that it wouldn't have gotten malignant, isn't that right?" My voice was going up again. "And if it was malignant a year ago, it *still* would have been better if they had taken it out right away. . . . I mean it sounds as if I was lucky that it didn't happen to spread. But it *might* have spread. It might have spread in that year and killed me. Isn't that right? *Isn't that right?*"

Larry's head was down. He folded his hands. "Of course it would have been better if they removed the tumor a year ago," he said, in an even lower voice than before. "They made a mistake. They were wrong."

"Why . . . why did they . . . make a mistake?" I whispered, knowing how stupid the question was.

He looked at me. "Because doctors make mistakes sometimes." That was the right answer, the only answer. But it was not the answer I wanted to hear. I bent over and held my stomach.

I did not want to know that doctors made mistakes. Doctors were like parents. I had always trusted them. I especially did not want to know that they had made a mistake on me. "I can't stand to know that," I whispered. "I know it happens, I know worse mistakes have been made—that's what all those lawsuits are about, but I can't stand it anyway." I looked up. "I can't stand it," I said, "because it's me.

"Larry"—my voice was gone, but I couldn't stop —"tell me more about the eighty-five percent. Where—where does that number come from? I know they're only numbers, I know they're *good* numbers. . . ." My hands were cold again. I clasped them, unclasped them, put them on my face, clasped them again. "I mean I know people with leukemia have worse numbers, much worse, awful, I mean I know when it's more than fifty, it's lucky, it's good, but—"

"I can't take this any more." That was Arthur.

The whole time he had been sitting on a chair opposite us, smoking and not saying a word. He got
up. "I'm going to work." He started to move
toward the study.

"Arthur," I said, louder than was necessary. He
turned around. "Please don't go. Stay here. I'll
stop soon, I promise."

"I just can't take it any more," he said, looking
down at the rug, and walked out.

I looked at Larry. "I can't help it," I said to him.

"I know," he said. "It's all right." Then he told
me what the percentages meant. "It just means that
there is a very good chance—an eighty-five-percent
chance—that there won't be a recurrence. And after
two or three years, if there is no recurrence, chances
are you're safe."

"You mean, if it's going to happen, it happens
soon?"

"Generally yes, within a couple of years."

"Oh, Larry, thank you."

He got up. "It's OK." And he left.

The wound hurt. It burned. And my arm ached.
The fact was I had less pain now than in the hospital, but the pain hadn't bothered me there. Nothing had bothered me in the hospital. I was asleep
then.

I wasn't asleep any more.

Death day wasn't over. After Larry left, I tried
to read, couldn't, tried to sleep, couldn't, until fi-

nally it was time to cook dinner, and I managed that. I'm a lousy cook—worse, an uninterested cook —so although I did it, I couldn't get lost in it, and in the middle of drying the lettuce, I started to cry again. The typewriter was still going in the next room. I didn't dare go in. Anyway, if I were to go in, what would I say? I had said it all. Now I had to bear it.

But that was the problem. What do you do when you can't bear it? There is only one thing *to* do: Bear it. Later, some people, some women, would ask me, How could you bear it? Answer: You bear it, because what else are you going to do? What are the alternatives? Not to bear it? What does that mean? You bear it, because not to bear it is to crack or to kill yourself. One can't *choose* to crack—you do or you don't—so that is not an alternative. To kill yourself is, but who would be crazy enough to do that?

I knew this as I dried the lettuce, but I also knew I was not off to a good start. There must be a bearing-it technique that I didn't know about. I couldn't go back to my act. And I couldn't keep bugging people. Even if they were nice about it, I couldn't keep that up. And, clearly, Arthur had had it—at least for now.

I was angry at Arthur. I knew I shouldn't be, but I was. I knew it was awful for him, too. I knew that the relatives of sick or dying people have their own hell, and that sometimes it is a more barren,

103

lonely place than the hell of the person directly hit. I was perfectly aware that Arthur shared the horror of my illness without sharing any of the rewards. He suffered and he was afraid, but no one pitied him, visited him, brought him presents, or made him a star. Stardom in a hospital bed was small compensation for having breast cancer, but it was, as they say, better than nothing. At least it gave me the right to be temperamental. Arthur didn't even have that. On the contrary, he was supposed to be perfect.

I expected him to be perfect. And I was furious when he wasn't. And I was furious with myself for being furious at him. And I couldn't help it. I throbbed with feelings I knew I shouldn't have: rage, self-pity, fear, frailty. I didn't like myself for having them. I liked myself in the hospital better. I liked that phony in the hospital, that Sleeping Beauty. She was good. She was cheerful. She was brave, a good sport. Everyone loved her. Who would love her now? Even her own husband was (understandably) turning against her. Where did she go, that Good Betty? I stood at the sink and thought about her. I also thought about the other Good Betty—Mrs. Ford, waving gamely with her bad arm from the White House balcony—and those other brave, good ladies. "Just fine," Happy Rockefeller had said, when a reporter asked her how she felt after her mastectomy.

And what of those other good, smiling, brave,

famous ladies? Fine, they were all fine. "I'm happier than I've ever been in my life," beamed Marvella Bayh on syndicated television after her operation. What was the matter with me? I was one of the lucky ones, after all. No bad stuff in the nodes. Why was I being such a lousy sport all of a sudden?

I wanted to kill Smith. Smith and Ellby together. I wanted to kill them both. I thought about what Smith said about "primitive" medicine. "Primitive, my ass," I should have said. "What if I were your wife? Would you have let your wife sit around for a year with a lump, a hard, cancerous lump? Would you? Would you?" I screamed at him in my head. But that was the only place I screamed at him, because I never saw him again. I never saw Ellby again either. But Larry saw him and asked him about my case. Larry reported back to me what he said: "Well, we're right ninety-six percent of the time."

Months later, I talked about the treat-me-like-your-wife notion with a friend who is a doctor's wife. "That's exactly how Bob treats all his patients," she said. I wondered. Even with good intentions, can a doctor—can a person—really do that? Is it fair to expect that? Can anyone maintain such a high level of concern? Furthermore, is the treatment a doctor gives his wife necessarily the best kind of treatment? Perhaps in treating a wife or child a doctor is too conservative. Does the wisest medical judgment necessarily come from love? Don't doctors sometimes send their wives and children to other doctors for treatment?

Other doctors. That's it, I thought. I couldn't fault Smith and Ellby for not recommending the removal of my lump if, in their best judgment, they didn't think it was cancer. "We can't remove every lump," Smith had said on the phone. But I came to realize what he and Ellby might have done, might have suggested, and what, I think, they would have insisted upon were I a wife or a child. As long as there was any doubt as to what the lump was—and there had to be some doubt—they should have sent me to another doctor, to Singermann. That idea is neither new nor novel. My mother even has a maxim for it: "Always get another opinion," she says. Right again, Mom.

The typewriter in the next room was still going at full speed. I got up. I am lucky, I told myself, as I walked into the bathroom and swallowed another Valium. I am lucky. If cancer was in my body for a year it seems to have stayed in one place. But it might not have. It might have spread. It might have killed me. It might still.

12

So: OUT OF THE HOSPITAL Sunday. Monday, death day. Tuesday, partial recovery from death day—a little less despair, a little more anger. And on Wednesday I went to a cocktail party.

It was at Joanna Simon's. Joanna had been one of the people on my S.O.S. list that weekend before surgery. She wasn't home when I called, it turned out, because she was in the hospital herself, with a broken hip. Nor was she well, yet, either. But she wanted to have a party, she said, because it was so boring to be laid up, and besides, it was her boyfriend's birthday. I wanted to go to the party because after three days of feeling rotten, a decreasing flow of visitors and flowers, and a husband who was losing patience, I longed for the good old hospital days. I couldn't get them back, but a party at least might help me revive my good old hospital *self*. Wow, three days out of the hospital and she's at a cocktail party. Whatta kid. Whatta woman. I could use a little of that. Also, I wanted to see if I could camouflage the war zone, if I could still get myself up to look nice.

It might have been the Senior Hop. I took an hour and a half to get ready. It took one third of that time just to find the right blouse, one that was loose enough. There wasn't much to pick from. Most of my blouses and tops were tight, because of the nice tits I used to have and because I used to show them off. But none of that. No looking back. No looking front, either! Ha-ha, joke.

I rigged up a fabulous bogus left breast for the occasion. What a clever girl. Here's how I did it: put on my loosest bra, hooked it on the loosest hook, so that it would go over the bandage, stuffed it first with Arthur's white tennis sock (too big), then a stocking (too small), then two stockings (just right). Then, off to the ball!

I was a sensation. OK, OK, so my entrance was a little wobbly. People just thought I was coming from another cocktail party. But I talked, I giggled. I did my nice-to-see-yous and fines in response to everyone's how-are-yous, but I kept wondering who knew, who knew and were pretending they didn't. The ones who said, What have you been up to? Haven't seen you on the tube lately—they, surely, didn't know, because they wouldn't have said that, right? It was easier with them, so I prattled on about the fascinations of teen-age alcoholism.

And as I talked and listened to myself, all at once I thought, My, it's old me talking, not even the hospital whatta-kid me, but the original me, the one Before. All because the people who talked to me didn't know and didn't see. Was that all it took? If somebody thinks I'm good old me, does that make me good old me? I had a drink.

"You've gotten so thin!" cooed a woman whom I knew slightly. She was being complimentary, of course.

Darling! I found something that beats Dr. Stillman's water diet and Kounovsky's exercises combined! Cancer! *Guaranteed* to take off a few pounds or the cost of surgery back! . . . "Thanks," was what I actually said.

I was drunk, but not so drunk that I didn't know I was passing. I *was* passing. Incredible. Nobody knew. Nobody could tell. They thought I looked wonderful. Thin. "Lovely," someone else said. Each time someone complimented me, I ducked into Joanna's bathroom and, standing on my toes, checked myself out in the medicine-cabinet mirror. Front and side. Then I repowdered my face and went back into the living room for another go.

Was this a feminist talking? Was I not a woman whose self-esteem hung on her personhood, rather than her looks? What was this perverse terror of *not* being a sex object? Was I, am I, not above that? Answer: No, I am not and have never been and probably never will be above that. Nor are most women I know, most of whom are ardent, authentic, card-carrying feminists. Sure, for a while some of them pretended to be above caring how they looked. Or they practiced not caring. (In the late sixties, Lois Gould didn't wear eye makeup for a year, and Gloria Steinem stepped into a pair of blue jeans and, as far as I know, never stepped out. Of course, Gloria Steinem looks good in blue jeans, a fact of which she must be at least minimally aware. One of the things I've always liked about Betty Friedan, incidentally, is that from the beginning of the women's movement, she—shamelessly—has never stopped going to the beauty parlor.)

The hope was, I suppose, that if you practiced not caring, you might stop caring. Erica and I used to rage against our mutual vanity investments; Erica wrote a terrific piece in *The Village Voice* (after it was rejected by *Ms.*) about the appalling amounts of both time and money spent on the upkeep of one's surface. Worse than a car, or even an apartment. This did not go for all women, we knew that, but it did for most of the women we knew—single or married—in New York. I used to think it would all stop after marriage, but it didn't. Vanity persisted like a tic.

When I was in the sixth grade, there was a contest at the end of the year: who was the most this, the best that. I was voted the smartest girl, but Lorraine Solzer was voted the prettiest, and (even though I came in second) I cried. Has nothing changed? Answer: Plenty has changed, but not that. Scratch most feminists, heterosexual or homosexual, and underneath there is a woman who longs to be a sex object. The difference is, that's not *all* she longs to be. If I were in the sixth grade today, I'd be happier than I was to be the smartest, and slightly less miserable about not being the prettiest. But only slightly. Most women I know have come to terms with their lingering sex-objecthood wish. For one thing they realize that wanting to be attractive and sexy is human—something that men want too, and nowadays more men are admitting it. There was a time when a scintilla of male vanity made a man seem—God forbid—effeminate. Not any more. So what has changed is merely that both men and women want to be the smartest and the prettiest now. As for me, I still felt ranked with the former; but as for the latter, as for the beauty contest: disqualified.

Everyone at the party thought I was still pretty. I passed, all right. But transvestites pass, too. It's nice to fool everyone. It's nice to get a prize for your costume. But it doesn't stop you from knowing, yourself, what's underneath.

I got a little drunker. Then we left the party and went home.

13

SINGERMANN HAD GIVEN ME some instructions. Since I had a shortage of infection-fighting lymph nodes, now and for the rest of my life, I was to avoid getting an infection on my left arm or hand. That meant, among other precautions, I was no longer to cut my cuticles. "But I bite my cuticles," I told Dr. Singermann. "Bite your right hand," he said.

He also gave me two exercises to do twice a day. The first was to face the wall, an arm's length away, extend my bad arm, and "walk" up the wall with my fingers until it hurt. I was to mark that place, and the next day move closer and go up a bit farther. The first couple of times I got about as high as my nose. After about two weeks, though, I was able to stand right up against the wall and go straight up. I wondered if retarded people feel the same way the first time they weave a basket.

The other exercise was to do the same thing, but sideways; that is, with my bad side to the wall, bad arm out to the side, and go up the wall that way. I hated the second exercise, because every time I did it, it felt as if my chest were splitting open. That

112

was silly, of course. All I felt was pull, and that was how the exercise was supposed to feel. Just the same, I dreaded it.

That wasn't all I dreaded. I dreaded going to bed. In the first place, I couldn't get comfortable in bed, which meant I couldn't fall asleep, even when I took a Valium. The pain wasn't bad, but I was sore enough not to be able to sleep on my front or on my left side, which, as it happens, were the two places on which I had always slept. Wouldn't you know. Sleeping on the right side didn't work well, either, because that meant my left arm rested on my left side. It helped to put a pillow under the arm, but that was awkward and uncomfortable, too. So I slept on my back, which made me feel like a corpse. I knew this was all very minor, passing stuff. None of it had bothered me in the hospital. But in the hospital, nothing had bothered me.

Another reason I dreaded going to bed was that I dreaded sex. "It's not you, it's me," I'd say to Arthur.

"It's OK," he'd say. But I could tell it wasn't.

"This won't go on forever, you know," I'd say to his back. But I knew he thought it might. And the truth was, I wasn't sure myself. What the hell was wrong with me? Wasn't this all backward? I should think he wouldn't want *me*. I just was not having the kind of sexual problems that I thought I was supposed to have, the ones I had heard and

113

read about. I did not worry that my husband would no longer find me attractive. He found me attractive. He wanted me. The crazy thing was, I did not want him. He still found me attractive, all right, but I did not. I no longer found me attractive. I was damaged goods now, and I knew it. It had begun to dawn on me, as other things had begun to dawn on me, that underneath the bandage was something very ugly. I didn't know yet how ugly. But I didn't have to. It was enough to know that I was mutilated, a deformed person. If you feel deformed, it's hard to feel sexy. For me, anyway, feeling sexy had a lot to do with feeling beautiful, or at least whole. Those narcissistic feelings were short-circuited now. The fuse had blown. And with it, my sex light went out. I was dark and dry. I no longer felt lovely. Ergo, I no longer could love. Simple as that.

My third dread in bed was dreams. Bad dreams. One morning, after three successive nights of these, I wrote them down:

A young, handsome doctor is examining me. He touches my breast; then he moves his hand to the other side. He leaves his hand on the flat place and looks at me. He says nothing, but his look is sexy and tender. He leaves his hand there and continues to look at me that way. But I can't stay. I get up to leave, and I know that I won't see him again.

I am a child and I have lost my arm. I must wear a horrid, pink, plaster-of-Paris thing, like the arms of my dolls. But my dolly's arms have fingers, and mine has none. So I must also wear a hook. Like hideous, bad Captain Hook in Peter Pan. I start to cry. I sob. The sobbing wakes me up.

I am on a train. There is a club car on the train filled with men in suits. In the club car there is a bathtub with a curtain around it. But one can see through the spaces between the sections of the curtain. I want to take a bath. I know that the men in the club car might be able to see me in the bathtub, but I want to take a bath anyway, because, although I don't admit it, even to myself, I want them to see me. I want to show off my body— especially the prettiest part of me, the part that shows when one sits up in a bathtub: breasts.

In order to take the bath, one must make certain arrangements. I need to tell a porter, and I need certain equipment—a washcloth and a shower cap. I am unable to find a porter, and I can't seem to find a washcloth and shower cap. There are other vague obstacles—I cannot remember what they are —to my taking the bath. But finally the way seems clear. I have not done everything or found everything I need to do and have, but I do have a washcloth and almost everything seems in order. Then I hesitate. There is something else in the way that is stopping me. I can't figure out what it is. Then I remember what has happened to me. I remember that there is nothing to show off about any more. I no longer want the bath.

I went back to my ex-psychoanalyst, Dr. Rumfeld, who made me feel better about not wanting sex. "You're in mourning," he explained in the same German lilt I had heard lying on his black leather couch with a paper napkin under my head from 1963 to 1967. "You have had a death in the body."

A death in the body. Rumfeld had the nicest way of putting the most God-awful things. And his literary analogies—all German—were lovely. For years I was this Mann character, or suffering from that Goethe feeling. It gave a certain breadth to one's mundane difficulties.

It was odd being there. I felt like a former student coming back to the old professor for a graduate seminar. Part of my new status was that I sat up in a chair, like him, and talked to his eyes, instead of to the ceiling as I used to do, or to the George Grosz painting on the wall opposite. When I got over the thrill of being eyeball to eyeball, though, my eyes moved away from his—to the window, where I could see the sky and the soft tops of greening trees in Central Park. I wound up talking half to him and half to the trees.

We talked about a lot of things: my marriage, my mother, my past, old torments, and, now, the new one.

I had forgotten how good it was to spill and, no matter how vile, to have one's spillings accepted with equanimity and intelligence. Psychoanalysis is no longer stylish and almost no one can afford it, but I feel about it the way some people feel about other wonderful luxuries of the past, like fresh whipped cream or Paris. I'm glad—intensely and humbly glad—I was able to swing it when I did.

Psychoanalysis made me happier and smarter. It also made it easier to be honest. Because, if analysis works, you find out that the awful truths about yourself are not so awful. At the very least, you find out they're not original. If *you* are a louse, you grow to think, so is everyone else. That is debatable, of course, but if you buy it, you wind up liking yourself more, which, in turn, makes you both less of a louse and less of a liar. Because the more you like yourself, the less you hide the truth about yourself.

There is another kind of help for women who have had mastectomies. The American Cancer Society sponsors a program called Reach to Recovery, started by a woman named Terese Lasser, who had a mastectomy in 1952, pulled herself out of a severe depression, and decided to help other women in the same boat. Now there are about two thousand volunteers in Reach to Recovery—most of whom have had mastectomies themselves—who do what they can to help "newcomers." They visit women in the hospital after surgery and give them everything from reassurance (I-had-it-and-I'm-OK sort of thing) to practical assistance and information about exercises and what to do about clothes.

It sounded like a fine idea, but even so, I opted not to see a volunteer. I guess it sounded clubby to me. I have never been clubby, and I wasn't about to start by joining a cancer club. I had no wish to see "another one." Besides, I had Rumfeld and the telephone.

During that first week at home, I kept swinging up and down. Mostly down. I had not figured out any new techniques for handling the downs, except to keep talking and, occasionally, writing. A few more people knew what had happened to me now, so there were a few more ears to bend. As I got stronger, I invited people to lunch. Anyone who came paid dearly for their eats. It was one tuna fish sandwich in exchange for an hour of Betty and her breast.

Sometimes I reverted to my brave act. But mostly not. Mostly I just yammered. I said the word a lot: cancer. I liked to say it, I needed to spit it out. That was hard on some people, I know. Doctors aren't the only ones who prefer "malignancy" or "mammary carcinoma" to cancer. People who come for lunch don't like it much either. Even the women I know who say "fuck" wince at "cancer." The technical words, I guess, sound safer. They're more distant, less personal. "Malignancy" sounds like something that happens to a cell. Most people can't picture a cell. Or if they can, they picture it as a thing. Cancer, on the other hand, sounds like something that happens to a person. A person like you, maybe.

In the same spirit, I much preferred "breast-cut-off" to "mastectomy." Mastectomy, like malignancy, is not only more distant, it also has a rather official sound—like something you salute.

Anyway, people don't like "breast-cut-off" any more than they like "cancer." Breast-cut-off is too active, too descriptive. Breast-cut-off says what happens. And who wants to hear that, especially over a tuna fish sandwich? Why did I need to say it? I'm not sure. In a way, it was like vomiting. Perhaps I thought that if I kept spitting up I'd get rid of it and feel better. I did feel better. But then I'd feel worse almost right away again. So more throwing up. And more feeling better. And more feeling worse.

I was big and brave with the words, but I wanted nothing to do with the reality of that place on my body. I was like one of those governmental welfare policy makers who can't stand the actual sight of a poor person. What saved me were not meetings and written reports but my bandage. Thank God, in those early days, for the bandage. It was not only a screen which hid the disaster area; it was also, in a way, prosthetic. The bandage was padding. It stuck out some, so it lessened the difference between the two sides—the side where there was a small breast and the side where there was nothing at all. Not that I looked myself over much. Screened or not, I did my dressing and undressing fast, eyes front, and I kept away from mirrors.

Bathing was troublesome, because taking a bath meant being naked for at least five minutes. Nor could I hide from myself in the water, because I could only bathe from the waist down, so as not to wet the bandage. There was also the problem of having to wash the remaining breast, which I learned to do without looking down. There were moments when, in order to wash carefully around the bandage, I did have to look down, but I developed a technique for that, too. It was an attitude, really—more role-playing. I pretended I was a nurse and that the body I was washing was someone else's. I was thereby able to assume a certain perfunctory attitude while washing around my deformity and, at the same time, in a thoroughly businesslike and efficient way, do the job.

One reason I looked forward to my first appointment (and subsequent ones) with Dr. Singermann, four days after getting out of the hospital, was that there was a real nurse there. It was sublime to lie on an examination table and be a patient again. Arthur and my mother had taken turns attending to my nonmedical needs the first few days at home. But it wasn't the same. I wanted chilly, professional attention. I wanted to be handled by people who made me feel routine, normal. People who were used to the likes of me and my body.

The nurse wasn't the only turn-on during those early Singermann visits. There was also the doctor. My in-hospital romance with David was platonic

120

compared to what I suddenly felt for, of all people, Dr. Singermann. At first I thought I had those feelings because he was objectively devastating and I had been too upset before to notice. I passed over his age, sixty-three (I had a friend look him up in a medical directory), and his walleye as endearing imperfections. I saw only how lean he was, how elegant, how—enigmatic. I saw him as a man who feels more than he shows. Among his hidden feelings I imagined was his (barely controllable) passion for me. Not that I thought it was just sex he wanted, or that it was just sex I wanted from him. I am a fifties girl and my sexual fantasies are, at bottom, domestic. In my dreams we not only screwed, we had dinner parties. I did not ignore his wife; I thought of her often—as an elderly blur in a suit, dried up enough not to mind if I took her husband away from her. His children, I reasoned, were grown and they wouldn't mind either. And that was that for any guilt I might have had (which I didn't).

Why did I lust for my dear, elderly surgeon? Because during those weeks he was the only man with whom I felt beautiful. He was used to the sight of severed breasts. He created them, for God's sake. And in his land of one-breasted women—mostly, I assumed, older and saggier than me—I felt like a goddess. Mirror, mirror, on the wall, I was the prettiest freak of all. Freud calls that feeling narcissistic. Feminists say it's at the bottom of sex objecthood. Whatever it is, and whether or not it would be better not to have that feeling, I have that feeling. In order to feel attrac*ted,* apparently I have to feel attrac*tive.* And the only man who made me feel that way (not because of anything he did, of course, only because of my madness) was old walleyed Dr. Singermann.

Meanwhile, for my poor husband I remained dry as a gourd.

14

On Saturday night, I rigged myself up for another social event. I put on the same bra I had worn to Joanna's, shoved the same pair of stockings into the left cup, pulled on the same baggy black over-blouse, and went off with Arthur to a dinner party uptown.

It was awful. First of all, the hostess had a cleavage which looked like the Mitla Pass. Since she opened the door and was, therefore, the first person I saw, the evening soured right away. Dinner was good, and I had a perfectly pleasant time talking to some of the other guests. But my eyes were like a Frisbee. No matter whom I talked to and where else I looked, I kept coming back to Mary's cleavage. Funny thing is, Mary is short and what used to be called top-heavy. God knows, I never wanted to be top-heavy. Even when I was thirteen, I never wanted breasts that big. But I wanted them now. They did make me slightly queasy, and the more I looked, the queasier I felt still, but I couldn't stop looking.

No one in this group knew what had happened

to me, either. I liked that the first time around at Joanna's. But this time I felt alone with a bad secret. At one point, I thought I might just tell someone, anyone. But it was one of those chitchatty, cozy dinners-for-eight, and there was no opening, no possible way to say cancer or breast-cut-off or even breast, so I gave up and ate a lot of chicken and drank a lot of white wine.

Then, two evenings later, things picked up again. Larry Cohn came over with Judith Ramsey, another friend who knew, and I bought an enormous lasagna from a new takeout place and I got some overpriced but altogether wonderful endive from the overpriced market on Second Avenue, and we had a perfectly swell time.

By the time my next appointment with Singermann rolled around the following Thursday, I was in something approaching good spirits, and the appointment itself revved me up even more.

My mother met me at Singermann's office. We had decided it was time for my reentry to Bloomingdale's, and we sat down in the waiting room and talked about where else it might be fun to go— Bendel's, maybe.

As we talked, I noticed two women across the room. One was about fifty. She had a nice, rumpled look and a noticeably large, hooked nose. The other woman, about twenty-five, had the same nose and was obviously the first woman's daughter. They were both very still. Except for occasional heaving sighs from the mother, neither one made a sound or even moved. They were both very obviously and very seriously distraught.

After a few minutes I got up and asked the receptionist how long a wait there would be. I was next, she said, explaining that the other young lady was here for the first time, so that meant a long appointment, and rather than keep me waiting that long the doctor would take me first. I thanked her and sat down and looked again at the girl and her mother. I noticed how thin they were. They looked as if they were losing weight from terror on the spot. (Isn't it curious, I said to my mother later, over tea in Schrafft's, here *they* were, not really knowing, only suspecting this awful thing might happen, and here *we* were, having *had* the awful thing happen, and we were, by far, the cheerier pair. My mother listened carefully, then put down her teacup and pulled out the appropriate sampler, which as usual was on target. "Fear," she said, "is the worst.")

The nurse called me to the examining room. I smoothed down my skirt and wet my lips.

This appointment was an almost exact repeat of the last one: another bandage change—eyes front as always—another exercise lesson, and, incredibly, even more thrills and chills than last time, brought on, of all things, by my fears of shaving my left armpit. The underarm of that side was still completely numb, and shaving a numb armpit was not only creepy but, in view of the danger of infection, terrifying as well. Singermann had told me to shave and just be careful. But I couldn't do it. I did the right arm and started the left, and the combination of seeing a razor blade against my skin when there was, at the same time, absolutely no sensation gave me a chill.

"What's this?" said Singermann, when he noticed what I hadn't done.

"It's a hairy armpit. Whaddya think it is?" I shot back. Then, in a slightly nicer tone of voice, I explained why I hadn't shaved.

He sighed. "Do we still have a razor somewhere around here?" he said to the nurse.

"I'll look for it," she mumbled, with something less than consummate interest.

"Oh, for Christ's sake," I said, "you *don't* have to shave my armpit!"—thrilled, of course, at the prospect.

"Ahh," he said with his sexy half-smile, "I haven't done my good deed yet today."

I wasn't crazy about that remark, but I wasn't going to let it spoil what lay ahead. "Here," said the nurse, handing him an old-fashioned steel razor with obvious disapproval. Gently, he raised my arm and soaped it slightly, and gently, with tender and absolute concentration, he shaved me.

I shut my eyes. Nobody spoke. A little more soaping, a little more shaving. So precise! So sweet! So sure! So pornographic!

The two stockings didn't work. Stockings have no weight, and breasts do, so I was always off kilter.

126

If I raised my arm, which I now was able to do, the left side of the bra with the stockings would rise, and when I lowered my arm the weightless buggers would stay up. Also, the stockings looked funny. They were lumpy. And my loose-fitting shirts were not that loose-fitting.

So I decided to have a look at a place Singermann told me about where they sell false breasts. Naturally, they're not called that. They have one of those nice, distant, more-than-two-syllable names: prosthesis (singular); prostheses (plural).

The place, which turned out to be in an office building, was started by a woman who had It. My stomach tightened as the elevator went up. It had suddenly occurred to me that I might be in for a horror show: a crowd of women who looked like me.

There was only one. As soon as I opened the door, I saw a woman about my age, standing on her toes, showing a man—her husband, I assumed—a swimsuit she was trying on. It didn't look like a swimsuit. It looked like a leotard. That's because it went clear up to the neck and it had cap sleeves. My God, will I have to wear one of those? Then I thought, No, probably not, because I still have a chest—that is, a chest muscle—so I don't really have to cover up all of that, just the part where the breast was. I think.

I looked at the face of the woman. She was smiling—rather coyly—turning this way and that, much to the approval of her husband, who sat on a bridge chair with her purse in his lap. It might have been outside a dressing room at Saks or some other normal place. The whole shop did, in fact, look "normal"—like one of those small women's specialty shops on Main Streets in small towns.

There were clothes racks with nightgowns and bathing suits. Most of the bathing suits had peculiar, covered tops, but that was not noticeable at a glance. Behind the counter, ceiling to floor, there were shelves with white boxes, the kind that usually hold slips or underpants. It was not at all obvious what the boxes did hold. The two saleswomen were both busy at the other end of the store, so I peeked into one of the boxes. There, in cellophane, with white tissue paper around it, was a single, rounded, pinkish blob, about six inches wide, four high, and three deep. It was a breast. I closed the box.

The rest of my visit to the shop is a blur. A saleswoman finally came over and told me it was too soon after surgery to get one of the things in the box (which I did not ask to see again). She sent me off with a temporary prosthesis—a four-dollar wad of Dacron, which looked like cotton, with a flesh-colored nylon cover, and I got out of there fast.

That was my first dip into the land of phony breasts. It was a month before either the outer me or the inner me was ready for the second.

15

ON MONDAY, April 22, eight days out of the hospital, I had gone back to work.

Or, I should say, I had gone to the office. Nobody sent me out to cover any race riots, or even any press conferences. They all thought (and said) I was crazy to be there that soon, and, of course, I was. My chest still burned, my arm ached, and since I was still bandaged, I was, to say the least, not agile. Not that it would have mattered. Thanks to my lingering anemia, I had almost no energy.

So I sat at my desk like a drunk on a stoop. And people sort of walked around and over me. Let her sit there, she's not bothering anybody. But, I had reasoned, if I went back to my normal life, I'd feel more normal. So I did what I could: fiddled with film, cut the *Ms.* magazine piece, and took a look at teen-age alcohol. Four producers had fooled around with it while I was gone, which meant that it had been cut up and put together again four different ways. The film editor was sick of it, as well she should have been. It was a mess. I heard it ran sometime during that following summer. I never saw it.

Going back to work didn't work. First, I did not feel like my normal self, as I had expected to. I felt strange, and I felt exhausted. The exhaustion annoyed me and the strangeness depressed me. The latter had to do with other people. At a place like NBC News, where people are constantly flying off to other continents for indefinite periods of time, a two-week absence is hardly noticed, so most people didn't miss me and didn't know. That was fine, but I didn't know for sure who knew and who didn't. And that made me uneasy.

The people in my own bureau (a bureau chief, three other correspondents, three field producers, a news director, and a secretary) had been among the flower-and-card senders, so I knew *they* knew. On my first day back, they greeted me with massive warmth—affectionate cheek kisses and hand squeezes—all of which pleased and touched me. But I had another reaction to their kindness.

Clearly they felt sorry for me, and although I still fancied pity from individuals, a group pity scene got me down. Part of that, again, was the contrast. I was used to being utterly unpitiable. One reason was that, just before the operation, my career was blooming. Nobody was sending me to Washington to cover the White House, but I didn't want to be sent to Washington to cover the White House. I was doing what I liked to do: long features about trends and such, as opposed to news events. They were good pieces, too. And besides my work, there was my generally "up" frame of mind. Although I was not thoroughly and deeply happy, I was thoroughly and deeply cheerful, and that showed; indeed, I had a lot to be thoroughly and deeply cheerful about, and people knew it.

So people had related to me in terms of my good fortune, and suddenly to be related to in terms of my bad fortune was strange and somewhat dismal. With those who knew, I tried to be funny about it —I told about all those tits in all those boxes—and people laughed, but they laughed with a kind of sorrow, which of course was part of their affection for me, and I appreciated it, but it made me feel sorrowful, too.

Moreover, everybody else seemed so un-tired. And young.

On Friday of my second week back at work I had an appointment with Singermann that I dreaded. The bandage was due to come off. I had made the appointment late in the day again, so it wouldn't interfere with all the work I wasn't doing. I figured I might not be good for much afterward. I tried not to think about it during the day and almost succeeded. An hour before the appointment, which was at five o'clock, I was jumpy enough to take a Valium—the first in several days.

Just as I was leaving NBC, the sky got very dark and it began to thunder. I got into a taxi. By the time I arrived at Singermann's building, it was pouring. My mother had suggested that both she and my father meet me there this time, and afterward they would drive me home. "OK," I said, and when I got there, they were already in the waiting room. There were no other patients, and I was called into the office right away.

I took off my blouse, as usual, and put on one of those paper gowns and sat there for a moment with my feet dangling off the examination table. Then Singermann came in. He was wearing his white coat, as usual, and a beautiful silk pastel tie. "How are *you?*" he said, brisk as usual. He never called me by my name—any name. For obvious feminist reasons, I had always resented doctors whom I addressed as Dr. So-and-so calling me Betty, but I wished Dr. Singermann would call me Betty. Especially that day.

He unwound the bandage and took it off, as usual, and, as usual, I kept my eyes straight ahead. But this time there was no new one wound immediately in its place. He gave the bandage to the nurse, and she pushed open the wastebasket—no!—and threw it in. My heart thundered inside my chest wall. There it goes, I thought. It was like watching a friend jump off a cliff. I lay down on the table, as I was told. With a small wet cloth, the nurse cleaned off the remains of the adhesive.

"You know," I said to Singermann, finding my voice, "I've never looked. I guess I better, huh?"

"Would you rather I left the room?" he said.

132

I looked at him. Not on your life, I thought, remembering the first time in his office when I collapsed and he had left the room then. I looked back up at the ceiling. "No," I said. Then I moved my eyes down the wall, to the sink, to the garbage disposal, to the bottom of it where my bandage was, to my feet. Then I lowered my chin and raised my head a few inches off the examination table and looked. I remember making some sort of sound. A moan, I suppose. Then I let my head fall back on the table. "Oh, God," I said. "Oh, God."

On the left half of my chest, where a breast had been, was a flat, lumpy surface like the ground, covered with, instead of dirt, skin. Across the surface, a long, horizontal, red, puffy welt meandered crazily from the center of my chest, where a cleavage once was, to the other side, under the arm, and around toward the back.

And alongside this little Hiroshima of the torso, on the unbombed half, grotesque by contrast, lay a right breast, pretty and whole as a healthy baby.

That was all I could take the first time around. Four days later I made myself take a second look, much in the same spirit as I sometimes make myself watch the torture parts in a movie.

It was after a shower. After drying myself I dropped the towel and stood square in front of the mirror. As a kind of preparation, I looked at the rest of me first. Face, eyes, neck, skip down to thighs (wish my legs were better, now the rest of me is messed up), belly (nice belly), and finally, for about thirty seconds, during which time I did not swallow, I stuck my eyes on the place of demolition. This is more than just an empty place, an empty lot. Destruction has happened here. Razed for development. Razed for no development. The scar is one track of a maniac's train, going nowhere. Not true, exactly; it goes to my back. Crossing the length of the track, every half inch, are short (one-inch) lines, not as crooked as the main line. These are the stitches. They are red, too, and swollen and very, very ugly. I want very much to look away now, but I don't. I let my eyes wander about the lumpy terrain and think about how they tell boys and girls apart. I think about the girl who was shot out of a cannon and no one believed that a girl would do that and so the next time she got shot out, she took her blouse off and then everyone knew she was a girl. Because girls have breasts. I cover my pretty right side with my hand and now there is just the left and I smile. It's sort of a joke: I don't look like a boy, after all. Even boys have nipples.

16

CLOTHES WERE my only screen now. I got to be a very fast dresser. When I put on my bra, I was especially speedy. I'd pin the prosthesis into the bra before I put it on. That saved me from having to look down to pin it in afterward.

With no bandage, baths were even more of a problem, so I took them less often. And when I did bathe, I had now mastered the technique of washing myself without looking—not altogether like a blind person, because I used peripheral vision. When it came time to wash there, I would fix my eyes hard on a nearby place, like my stomach (never at the remaining breast), and in that way, out of the corner of my eye, I could see just enough to wash properly.

Before, except in the winter, I had always slept naked. I wore nightgowns now. I bought several new ones.

I no longer liked to be on the street at all. With the bandage off, I felt unprotected and unsafe there. I was especially afraid for the small bump that was my heart. My heart was so close to the surface now. There was nothing in front of it any more, no flesh to protect it from getting hurt. Once I had an old, beautiful watch, and the back came off so that all the fragile workings were exposed, and I remember carrying it to the watchmaker in my hand, wrapped in a tissue, terribly (and irrationaly) afraid that I would fall (I never fall and I didn't then).

On the streets, I was not afraid of falling, the way I had been when I carried my watch; I was afraid of people. I was afraid of people hitting me —there—especially teen-age boys, walking toward me from the opposite direction. If I saw more than two of them coming, I'd cross the street. Or I would turn toward a shop window and flatten myself against the glass and pretend to look in the window, until the group of boys—or the menacing person—had passed by. I did that once and found myself staring at a windowful of clingy Italian and French T-shirts, the kind I used to wear on my other body. They caught me off guard and I started to cry, which was embarrassing because I didn't have my sunglasses. After that, I stayed away from shops that sold T-shirts.

With the bandages off, I seemed to hurt more. Not all the time but more often than before. I felt short, stinging, stabbing pains. Mostly on the nipple. But there was no nipple. I felt pain where there used to be a nipple. I had heard about people feeling pain in a leg they have lost. They hurt, they look down, and there is no leg. Disconcerting. Once I did that. I was at home, and I felt a stab.

My nipple hurts, said one voice. You have no nipple, said the other. But it hurts, I can feel it! said the first. So I opened my blouse and looked. The second voice was right, of course.

Under the arm, I was still numb. Sometimes numbness is worse than pain, because numb is dead. Speaking of dead: now, with the bandage off, I had stopped thinking about the big death but I couldn't get my mind off the small one—Rumfeld's death-in-the-body notion. One morning, after a bad night, I wrote down some thoughts I had about that. It was the first writing I did about the operation, and, I suppose, it was the beginning of this book.

May 2. I am like a widow who doesn't get it at first. Then she wakes up the next morning and the place next to her on the bed is empty, the sheets still tucked in on the other side, the pillow high and plumped, and she gets it then. I look at the empty place on my body and I get it, too. I get it.

A death in the body is, in some ways, like the other kind. One remembers the dead fondly. Sometimes the dead person seems more virtuous and wonderful than he or she was. I remember my left breast with love, real love. How I took it for granted! Isn't that silly; of course I took it for granted. Who goes around thinking, Gosh, lucky me to have two breasts. Don't I take my other parts for granted? Do I actively and devotedly appreciate my arms, my legs, my working brain? No. Not even now.

Difference between body-deaths and person-deaths: a person gets buried or burnt, ashes scattered, out of sight. The dead part of the body is destroyed too, of course, but the empty space remains. A widow can fill her dead husband's closets with her own clothing; she can fill the empty side of the bed with another man. The live man might turn out to be a better person than the dead man. The widow might grow to love the new man more. But no live thing can replace a dead breast. Only something else dead that comes out of a white box in the tit store.

If nothing live can take its place, how then can I get out from under this death? How can I lose it, forget about it, if the space cannot be filled and if, next to the space, reminding me of what I have lost every time I look at it, or touch it or have it touched, is the twin? I hate my living breast. It's not only that it reminds me of the other one. I hate it because it looks stupid by itself, hanging there, one of a pair, lopsided and foolish and blatantly incorrect. One candlestick on one side of the table, one lion on one side of the entrance to the New York Public Library, one shoe, one glove, one foot, one hand, one breast. Oh, God, God, maybe I am going cuckoo. That wouldn't be bad. If I were really cuckoo, I'd go to a cuckoo hospital. Cuckoo hospitals are in the country. They have lawns and wooden armchairs and oak trees and kind nurses in white.

At the same time that I hated my remaining breast, I loved it fiercely, like an only child. Like the one son not killed in the war. And the more I loved it, the more afraid I was of losing it, too. This double set of feelings produced a double set of reflexes. I hated my breast, so I couldn't bear to look at it. And I loved my breast, so I continuously felt it to make sure it was all right (lumpless). But while I felt it I tried not to look at it. Singermann had assured me that, of course, he would keep a careful eye on me; I would come in every three months for two years and every six months for the rest of my life—or his. Still, twice a day I kneaded away. Each time I found no lump, I felt terrific. For a couple of hours. Then, later in the day, worry would build again, and I'd feel myself again and there wouldn't be anything there and I'd feel good again. For the next few hours. Until the next time or the next day.

Aside from my self-examinational tic, I ravaged anything and everything I could find in print on the subject. I even read about cancer of other places: lungs, vaginas, glands, wherever. I read and reread the research from my old breast cancer story, perversely lingering over the scary parts. "The problem is," says Dr. Ruth E. Snyder, of New York's Sloan-Kettering Cancer Center, "that there are two breasts. If a woman has cancer in one, she has about a ten percent chance of getting it in the other." (At this point, without taking my eyes off the page, I'd start feeling myself again.) "Studies of biopsy material and of the 'other breast,'" the piece went on, "have taught us that breast cancer

139

is multicentric. It doesn't start in a single cell and develop in one source. It is very probable that there are multiple areas of cancer in one breast, and that is why the opposite breast is a high risk."

After the inevitable self-examination that followed, I would worry that, even though I couldn't feel it, a lump was there. Hiding. In the middle somewhere. That was not altogether silly. There are, indeed, lumps that cannot be felt. It is hoped that mammography picks up those. But as I well knew, mammography wasn't perfect either.

During this entire period, I was on a sort of shuttle. Either I felt thoroughly miserable about the repulsive state of affairs on my chest, or I felt thoroughly terrorized by the worst that might be yet to come: the loss of the other breast, or death. There was one saving grace about this shuttle. If I went in one direction, I could not, at the same time, go in the other. When I was really repulsed by my wound, not a thought entered my head either about having two or being dead. And when my head was heavy with death, the unloveliness of my chest seemed trivial.

Speaking of one misery canceling out another, Arthur was first to notice this one: As a well-adjusted, integrated city female, I worry a lot about robbery and rape. Mostly rape. I have locks on the door. Three. And a chain. And when I am in my apartment, I lock all the locks and hook up the chain. After my bandages were off, Arthur noticed that I no longer did that. Until he asked me about it, I hadn't realized what I was doing—or what I wasn't doing. Then I figured it out. I was no longer afraid of being raped because, I thought, who'd want me now?

17

I WAS STILL GOING to the office during my crazy time, and going out at night, too. I don't think my craziness showed much. That was partly because I was writing more, now, and putting my craziness down on paper. That made it more possible to be sane the rest of the time. Sometimes I reminded myself of one of those people who goes berserk and kills fourteen people from a rooftop and afterward the neighbors say, "But he was such a quiet boy. So polite." Then they find this loony diary.

Now and then, I would slip. At the oddest times. One evening, for example, we went to a dinner party in Princeton. A lot of smart, elderly, distinguished types. Republicans. Not the sort you act peculiar with.

I was seated next to the historian Emmet John Hughes, who once wrote presidential speeches for Eisenhower. He asked me one of those and-what-do-you-do questions, and I heard myself say, "I had a breast cut off recently, and I'm trying to get over it."

"Oh," he said, as the hand holding a fork froze midway between his plate and his mouth. This was not like the early spilling I did with friends; Emmet Hughes was not my friend. I didn't know what this was. Nor, poor man, did he.

In *Widow,* Lynn Caine writes that, during her crazy period, she once unloaded the fact of her husband's death on someone sitting next to her on a bus. I had heard of other people spilling both their miseries and their joys into the nearest (unknown) human receptacle. But why? To shock? Partially. It is heady to watch a person's hand freeze on the way to his mouth.

Also, to avoid feeling lonely. I had felt lonely at a party the week before. I didn't want to feel that way again. I wanted to tell. It made me feel less crazy to tell. There was so much craziness on my inside and so much normalcy outside, it was soothing to narrow the gap.

I didn't sock it to everyone. But when I did, once the shock was over, it usually turned out all right. Sometimes people responded to my news by disclosing cataclysms of their own, which were often as grim as mine or at least as interesting. Hughes, for example (after his fork found its way in and out of his mouth), swallowed and came forth with several intimate and arresting items about his life, his fear of death, and so on. This sort of exchange livened up a good many otherwise colorless social events.

That people who were spilled upon spilled back did not really surprise me. In my professional life, I had often both experienced and encouraged such behavior. When I wrote profiles for *Look,* one way I'd get people to show me their emotional innards was to show them some of mine. This was a sensible, successful, and, in a way, fair technique. It made the interview more of an exchange: I'll tell you if you'll tell me.

I never felt pressed to reveal that much. Most of the people I interviewed (movie stars and politicians) were monumentally narcissistic and had virtually no attention span, except a feigned one, for anyone else's inner life, no matter how juicy. So I never went on about myself—just enough to show that I wasn't judging them from a distant, protected place. It worked rather well. Rarely did I spill my beans and not get some back.

I told people about the mastectomy every time I felt like it. Although I hardly knew some of the people I told, I wouldn't tell anyone I didn't like. I told a lady at Kenneth who waxed my legs, a professor of mathematics at a cocktail party, and a saleswoman in the bathrobe department on the second floor of Bloomingdale's. I told Eugene. I told Beth Coolidge, a straight-talking and snooty-in-a-nice-way school chum from Boston whose response made my day: "My dear," she said in her most formidable lockjaw, "you will simply have to clutch one of those *attractive* little bags to your left side and *keep* it there." As solutions went, this was second only to Susan Wood's, who thought it would be nifty to get tattooed, "and then," she said, her mad, round little eyes lighting up behind her mad, round little glasses, "I'll photograph you *naked* for *Vogue*."

Not everyone had such innovative recommendations. Nor did everyone respond with a juicy story of his own. Nor did everyone respond in a nice way. Some people got pale and fled. Or they just fled. I understood that. If you are a victim, you can't expect to be popular. People don't like victims, especially unlikely ones. Victims like me give people a new, unpleasant sense of their own vulnerability. "Hey," they think, "if it could happen to her, it could happen to me." Who likes to be reminded of that?

Something else very crazy was going on during this time. While Arthur and I had stopped connecting almost altogether—in bed and everywhere else—my telephone romance with David was going like a warmed-up engine. He called almost every day, and if Arthur was around he would call back later. He told me he loved me, he told me he wanted to marry me, he told me again how he had always wanted to marry me and that he always thought he would—even after I married Arthur. I listened to all of this. I didn't know what to think, but I knew I liked it. I also knew I was scared. Guilty, too, but not very guilty. Once you've had cancer, I suppose you feel you have a right to be naughty. So I kept listening. Sometimes I'd think, This is crazy and bad and what am I doing? But I couldn't find the switch to turn it off. That was because I wasn't really looking for it.

It was not the first time in my life that I was out of control. But it was the first time I was willing to allow myself to be out of control. It was frightening. But I was even willing to be frightened.

Obviously, I was not going to keep my missing breast a secret, in spite of the warning from my sensible friend Helen Markel. She told me about another friend of hers who had had a mastectomy five years ago, and, said Helen, "She's fine now, but the one thing she regrets is that she told people."

When I heard that, it slowed me up some. For an entire day, I shut up. But I couldn't stand it. Besides, what did it matter now? I had already told half the world. Why not the other half? Moreover, I decided, I approve of telling people. It's good for the teller and the tellee. Why should humans hide their misfortunes from other humans, who are also vulnerable? Sooner or later, we all get hit. Why this macho pretense of invincibility? So some people get hit sooner and harder. So what?

Of course, it was easy to come clean about breast cancer now that the first and second ladies had done so. No question about it. The confessions of

146

Betty Ford and Happy Rockefeller and, before them, Shirley Temple Black and Marvella Bayh had made breast cancer socially acceptable. (One woman at NBC—a local reporter—actually came over to me in the hallway and said, "I hear you've got this year's chic disease.")

Just as the confessions of renowned homosexuals in public life made it easier for other homosexuals to "come out of the closet," so did the frankness of the first and second ladies help ordinary folks to open up. Even some prominent mastectomy victims, like Julia Child, did not "come out" until 1975, after about twenty years of hiding. One theory about why more women seem to have had the disease than ever before, by the way, is simply that more women *say* they have had it.

The new confessions made me wonder what it must have been like to hide, what it still must be like for the women who do. I knew one: Jacqueline Susann. Until she died, only her husband knew. I thought about how isolated and lonely I felt at just one party where no one knew. How could she bear it? But, obviously, for some people it is more bearable not to tell than to tell. Jackie Susann was a woman who frankly, openly, even blatantly loved her success. She was a winner (in society's terms, anyway: success, fame, money), and she wanted to be thought of as one. Losing a breast, again in society's terms and in hers, made her less of a winner. However screwy that may seem, if those are your

147

values, if that's how you feel, that's how you should act. Clearly, for Jackie Susann, a toppled image would not have been worth the relief of letting the secret out.

But even we who confess to our mastectomies nevertheless hide the way they look. Around the house, I didn't bother wearing the odious Dacron pad, but I wouldn't have dreamed of going out without it. Actually, sometimes, I did daydream about it, but that's all. Small-breasted or not, now that the bandage was off, there was a leviathan difference between the two sides of my chest that even the loosest, bulkiest clothes could not hide. That meant that if someone came to the door, or if I had to go downstairs to get a package, or if I was to confront anyone other than Arthur Herzog, my mother, or Dr. Singermann, I had to stick that thing on.

One day, about a week after the bandage was off, I had to make a fast trip to the corner market. (I was fooling around with a chicken-and-olives recipe and there weren't any olives.) Before my breast was cut off, I would have pulled on a pair of pants and a shirt and run out. But now I had to rig myself up in a bra so that I could stick the nylon thing in the bra (pinning it to the bottom so it wouldn't fall up and out); then, and only then, was I ready for a public appearance at the Italian market.

All of a sudden, the whole routine made me mad.

Dammit, I thought, why can't I go to the store for a can of olives with one side of me sticking out and one side not sticking out? Who the hell would care? But I couldn't do it. Because *I* cared. People might notice and I couldn't face that. I couldn't face the possibility of shocking and repulsing my fellow shoppers. In America, bodies are whole, teeth are straight, and the sight of a deformed person—that's you, kid—is a turnoff. It's unpatriotic to be a freak.

I remember the first time I ever saw a deformed person. I was about six, standing on a subway platform with my mother. There was a man nearby selling pencils. At first I noticed him because he was the only grown-up I had ever seen who was shorter than I was. The reason was he had no legs. He had stumps. When I saw the stumps I froze. The only people I had ever seen who were not perfect were monsters in books, and they were not real. Since this man was real, I knew it was wrong to feel the way I felt—somehow I knew he couldn't help it—but still I was nauseated. Our subway train came, finally, and my mother pulled me in. She asked me what was wrong. But I didn't know how to tell her, so I just shook my head and said nothing.

I thought about that incident when I went to the grocery store (wearing my apparatus). Clothed, I passed for normal. But it was strange to think that the sight of me undressed might frighten a six-year-old.

I thought about the subway incident again one

night when I pulled down the window shade of my bedroom before getting undressed. Pulling down the window shade is something I have done every night of my life since puberty, but now, I realized, I was doing it for a different reason. I was not pulling the shade down to keep the mythical Peeping Tom across the way from seeing my nice body, thereby tempting him to run over and rape me. I was pulling the shade to keep the mythical Peeping Tom from seeing my body and thereby throwing up.

18

THE PHONY TIT wasn't making it. I couldn't get the goddam thing to stay down. Even when I fastened it with a safety pin and lowered the left bra strap to zero, after a half hour or so the entire amalgamation rose like a buoy. It stayed down more when I hooked the bra tighter around me, but then it dug into the part of the wound that dipped under my arm, and that hurt. Also, the damn thing had no nipple. That wouldn't have mattered if my own remaining nipple didn't show, but God or whoever hands out nipples gave me a perpetually erect one. The only solution was a return trip to the tit shop to buy a proper made-to-order one-half-pound breast.

The second visit was, to be sure, less jarring than the first. But to my surprise and disappointment they did not sell—nor, they said, did anyone else sell—made-to-order prosthetic breasts. (That turned out not to be true.) They did have breasts in graduated sizes, however (like shoes!), and they were sure they could fix me up. The sales pitch amused me. Tits for sale: a business like any other.

I wondered if it went the same way in the leg-and-arm biz.

They did, indeed, have a prosthesis in my size. It was silicone and it was soft and pink and weighty. But it didn't have a nipple. Uh, I said, do you have one with a nipple? A nipple? they said. What an idea! They had no nipples, except for flat ones that were sort of drawn onto the form; nothing that stuck out. In a low voice I explained the problem of my idiosyncratically erect right nipple. The silence could not have been stonier had I announced syphilis. I picked up my Dacron wad, shoved it into my bra (without pinning it, so that by the time I got home it had edged up into the vicinity of my collarbone), and got out of there.

Swell, I thought. Wonderful. I was an outcast in the land of outcasts. I was not only a one-titted woman in a two-titted world, I was an erect-nippled one-titted woman in a flat-nippled one-titted world. I thought of a musical piece for children I had seen on television a few weeks earlier—Harry Nilsson's *The Point*—about a little boy with a round head who lives in a place where everyone has a pointed head, so they banish him to a forest where it doesn't matter if your head is round because no one else is there.

I called Reach to Recovery. Yes, they knew of a made-to-order place. In California. I called the man in California. Yes, he did make nipples. Yes, his "forms," as he called them, did have to be worn inside a bra, and yes, he would send me a brochure.

152

The problem was I had begun to do on-camera work again during the day; we were going out more at night. I felt that I could not go one more day without a nipple. Whereupon it occurred to me that perhaps I could make one myself—attach something small and pointed to the nylon cover of the Dacron wad. I headed for my sewing box, rummaged through spools of thread, buttons, pincushions, and cards of needles and pins, and there, in one corner of the box, under a green button, was a black nipple. Actually, it was a black cloth cuff link. But I knew right away it would work. I pulled up my blouse and held it next to my right nipple. Perfect. That is, the size and shape were perfect. The color, black, was not perfect. But what the hell. I wasn't planning to wear any see-through blouses.

Just as I threaded a needle and went to work, Arthur came home. "What are you doing?" he said.

"I just invented a nipple and I'm sewing it on," I said. "Now I know how Eli Whitney felt."

The next aim was to make it work without a bra. A few days later, I bought a role of surgical body tape and, with two strips on top and two on the bottom, taped my newly nippled prosthesis onto my body. Then I pulled on a T-shirt and looked at myself, first front, then side. It was magnificent. Really magnificent. I couldn't wait to show those harpies at the tit store—if I ever went back there again, which I probably would have to, to get a bathing suit. Meanwhile, it took a good deal of restraint not to pull my top up and show everyone I knew what I had wrought.

But I did restrain myself. The pride of invention was strong, but not as strong as the other feeling: the continual, reigning, omnipresent sense of being deformed. It turned me into something I had never been before: a modest woman. There is a boutique I used to like on Fifty-third Street. I walked in there one day—not very long ago—and walked straight out. I had forgotten about the group dressing room.

To hide in public seemed to me sensible and considerate. To hide at home was, I knew, something else. So far, only three people had seen me without a bandage: Dr. Singermann, Dr. Singermann's nurse, and myself. Sooner or later, Arthur would have to see me too. I couldn't keep hiding in my own house. I had sort of wished he had asked to see me, but he didn't. So one evening, while I was sitting in the bathtub, I asked him. "Arthur," I yelled.

"What?" he yelled back, from the other side of the bathroom door.

"C'mere," I said.

He opened the door slowly. The unwritten rule, since bandage removal, was that my baths were private. He peeked in. My left hand and arm were covering my left side.

"Wanna see?" I asked.

"Sure," he said, looking uncomfortable.

Suddenly, it didn't seem like such a good idea.

But it was too late. "Look," I said, and, keeping my eyes on his face, slowly I lowered my left arm.

He didn't flinch. "That's not so bad," he said. I shrugged. "It doesn't bother me a bit," he added, protesting a little too much.

"That's good," I said, slipping back under the water.

At a glance, the prosthesis brochure from California looked like something from a computer dating operation. MATCH-MATE, said the letters in big black type on a blue background, and, in smaller letters, Breast Prosthesis. Inside there was a drawing of a woman (wearing what I think was meant to look like a sexy dress) about to serve dinner to a man who was hovering over her adoringly. Restore Poise and Self-Confidence, dot, dot, dot, it said. And, on the other pages there were twenty Questions and Answers, e.g.: Q. Is the MATCH-MATE prosthesis filled with liquid? A. Definitely not! Accidental piercing of this type could be extremely embarrassing. Nor is MATCH-MATE the foam rubber type which can absorb perspiration and deteriorate. Farther down, it said that MATCH-MATE was made of a "special vinyl plastic" which is "chemically inert, which means it is not affected by body perspiration or other outside elements." (Like what, I wondered. Sleet and snow? Fire and water?)

It looked OK, but California was still a long way to go for a couple of ounces of vinyl. I decided to pay a call on Terese Lasser (the Reach to Recovery head) over at the American Cancer Society. Mrs. Lasser was reputed to know everything there is to know about prosthetic devices. On the phone, she had been first to confirm this. "If I don't know about it," she had said, "it doesn't exist."

Mrs. Lasser is an ample woman in her middle fifties and has what used to be called an imposing air. When I walked into her office, she was seated behind a big desk piled high with photographs, letters, and rubber breasts. The photographs and letters, which she showed me immediately, were of and from women who had had mastectomies. She held up one of the photographs—of a bride. "Isn't it wonderful?" she said. I agreed that it was wonderful and moved right on to the tale of my search for the perfect breast.

Before I got to the part about the nipple, she got up and went over to a cabinet on the other side of the room. "Try this," she said brightly, tossing me a pink blob that looked similar to the blobs from the tit store. No nipple. But it did have some weight. I looked at it more closely and gave it a squeeze. "It feels nice," I said, "but I think it's too big."

"I don't have a smaller one," said Mrs. Lasser. "Try it." I put it in my left bra cup. "Perfect," she said. It wasn't.

"Don't you think it's a little too big?" I asked meekly.

She sprang up again and pulled open another

drawer. She came toward me with some Dacron stuffing. "Try putting this in the other one." Obediently, I stuffed the Dacron in my right bra cup. "There, that's fine," said Mrs. Lasser, with a case-closed clap of her hands. (There were two other women waiting outside and someone else on the phone.) I gave myself a quick once-over in the full-length mirror on the back of her door. I was now bigger-breasted than I had ever been in my whole life. I thanked Mrs. Lasser—who, I felt, had done her best—put my own prosthesis in my purse, rounded my shoulders, and sped home, hoping I could get there without running into anyone I knew.

The next day I decided to try to improve the cuff-link-cum-nipple concept. Happily, there was a branch of the Singer Sewing Machine Company right in Rockefeller Center, very near NBC. After work I went over and headed straight for the button department. "Do you have any cloth buttons?" I asked a portly saleswoman with a permanent wave. No, she said, but here were the buttons they did have. There were hundreds, separated by color. I edged over to the tans and browns. This looks good, I said to myself, picking up a card of round, light brown buttons that looked soft. I felt one. It was plastic and not soft at all. There were some lighter brown ones nearby. They were also too hard and too big. The lady with the permanent wave was looking at me as if I were doing something dirty with her buttons. I moved away and found myself in front of the fringe counter. Wrapped around foot-high pieces of cardboard, there was enough fringe to hang the White House.

I stopped. On the bottom row, there were cards of ball fringe. Ball fringe. Balls. One of the fringes was a sort of golden brown. I zeroed in on the balls. They were the size of nipples and the color of nipples—well, maybe Oriental ones. Good enough, I thought, trying not to look too excited. I bent over and gave one of the balls a little feel. Soft as a cooked pea. I looked behind me. Permanent Wave was still staring. I straightened up. "I'll take that," I said with a show of authority.

She pulled out the card. "How much do you want?" she said, taking it over to the table yardstick.

I thought, I can't ask for one ball: "One quarter of a yard," I said.

She gave me a look. "The minimum we sell is a half yard."

"That'll be fine," I said. She rang up the sale; I handed her twenty-six cents and fled.

As soon as I got home, I pulled my sweater up for the old comparison test. Very good. Very, very good. I snipped off the cuff link with a nail scissors and sewed on the new nipple. It was gorgeous, absolutely gorgeous. There were seven more balls on the rest of the half yard that was left. Seven spares. I put them in my sewing box. Eight nipples for a quarter, I thought, feeling better than I had in days. Not bad.

When I went to take the prosthesis back to Mrs. Lasser, I noticed another woman outside her office, reading a magazine. She was about my age and pretty in a quiet, sweet way. Then my eyes dropped to her chest. She was wearing a T-shirt, and the difference in her breasts was so obvious I gasped. One breast was round and the other one was absurdly pointed. Unlike mine, her pointed one looked like the phony, not the round one. That was because the point didn't look like a nipple. It looked like the bottom of a paper drinking cup. Well, I thought, Mrs. Lasser will straighten her out.

Mrs. Lasser, meanwhile, motioned for me to come in and close the door. *"That* poor girl," she said, in a stage whisper. "She's only three weeks out of the hospital and her husband expects her to do *everything."* (She lingered meaningfully on the "everything.") "He's pushing her much too hard." I asked her what she meant. "He thinks the way to handle things is to push and she is very upset by it. I had a talk with him, but I don't know if it'll do any good." I said I was sure one of her little talks couldn't help but have an effect.

"How, by the way, are most husbands in this situation?" I asked her.

"Great," she said. "Mostly, it's the woman herself who is not so great."

The worst problem between husbands and wives, Mrs. Lasser went on to say, was misunderstanding. Sometimes the husband would try to be considerate and not press the wife about sex, for example, and the wife would interpret this as a loss of desire on his part. Or, she said, sometimes the husband would press too much. "But the biggest problem is not how their husbands feel about them, but how the women feel about themselves."

She stopped and looked at me. Then, seeing how interested I was, she went on. She knew women who couldn't bear to look at themselves—ever. She knew one woman who killed herself, another who slept in a separate bed from her husband the rest of her life. I asked her if a woman's age figured in her reaction to the operation. "Age has *nothing* to do with it," she said emphatically. "It has much more to do with vanity." The woman who killed herself was in her sixties. But she was an ex-opera singer and, in spite of her age, she thought of herself as being beautiful. When this thing happened to her, she simply couldn't take it. Of course, with extreme cases like that, there were always other problems as well.

"I better go now," I heard myself say to Mrs. Lasser. "Thanks for everything." Suddenly, I couldn't wait to get out. Although I found them engrossing, those stories did not have the same effect they had had on me when I was in the hospital. Other women's grief, now that I had experienced some myself, no longer cheered me up. On the contrary—although it was no fault of hers—Mrs. Lasser's tales depressed me the rest of that day and then some. I couldn't get the paper-cup woman's face out of my head. It's still there.

I took a bus uptown and another picture flashed into my head, the one of Betty Ford, waving on the balcony of the White House. I thought again of how much publicity there had been about those famous women and their bravery, and I realized more than ever how little publicity there was—none, really—about their dark days. Naturally (but why naturally?) if they had dark days they would have to hide them.

It was all very inspiring, those famous chins—up —but I wonder how many women might have been helped even more if they heard about the sad stuff as well. If I ever write about this, I vowed on the Third Avenue bus that day, I will tell about my sad stuff and let the other sufferers know they have company. And let the brave women feel braver still by comparison.

But for now I was on leave from the sadness and darkness. The prosthesis problem was, of course, a splendid distraction. Looking back, I'm sure that's largely why it became such an obsession. No doubt about it; the best way to stop worrying about something is not to try *not* to worry, or to focus on "something pleasant," but to work up a whole new worry about something *else*. The beauty of the breast hunt was that, unlike weaving baskets or pounding clay, it was not obviously therapeutic. At least not to me. As far as I was concerned, it was normal to spend most of one's waking hours thinking about breasts and detachable nipples.

Not that I was able to insulate myself completely

161

from dark thoughts and feelings. Sometimes they just snuck up from behind, like the reaction I had to Mrs. Lasser's stories. Other bad moments came like smacks in the back of the head. One day, for example, after my arm had more or less returned to working order, I decided to resume my calisthenics, which I used to do every day for five minutes and end by running in place one hundred times. I did not wear a bra when I exercised, so when I got to the running part I would always hold onto my breasts to keep them from bouncing. That day, after sit-ups and bicycle kicks, I began the final run-in-place and both hands went up, as they had always done, to hold my breasts. But in a couple of seconds my brain sent a reminder to my left hand that there was nothing for it to hold. I dropped my hand and kept on running, but I had to stop before reaching one hundred because I was crying too hard.

Months later, on a short holiday, at a pool in Key Biscayne, Florida, I was wearing my new prosthesis inside a specially sewn-in pocket in my bathing suit top (which was also stiched up an extra inch in the middle to hide the still puffy pink scar), so I no longer had the "prosthesis problem" to distract me. Time had gone by and it was a beautiful day and I lay on the deck chair with the sun high and hot overhead and my mind was far from the place on my chest where a breast had been. Then I looked up and saw a girl walk by in an extremely brief fuchsia bikini who began to strut, sort of, around the edge of the pool. She had very large breasts. I started to read, but every time I looked up I could see her sashaying back and forth toward the diving board and back and forth again. I tried to keep on reading, but she kept strutting and I kept looking up, and before I realized what had happened to me I was sobbing horribly. I had sunglasses, luckily, to hide my eyes, but no tissues, so I stumbled inside and ran up to the hotel room. It took about an hour before I was ready to leave the room, and I never did make it back to the pool.

That incident was no worse than several similar stabs of breast envy that had happened early on. But it hit me harder because it occurred when I no longer expected to feel that way. As I began to feel less awful about what had happened, I think I unconsciously expected it to "end"—the way my friend Joanna's broken hip had ended, the way most bad things I knew about ended. These incidents reminded me that, although I felt better about what had happened and would, no doubt, grow to feel still better, "what had happened" would never really end. Not ever.

After weeks of research, I finally went to Ann Arbor, Michigan, where, in the basement of the University's Medical Center, I was greeted by Denis Lee, a made-to-order prosthesis maker who swore he could make me a nipple that stuck out. From his name, I had expected him to be Chinese, but he wasn't. He was a sturdy young midwestern American whose father is a dentist. Mr. Lee's father's profession, it turned out, had no small bearing on his son's trade.

Mr. Lee's technique of prosthesis-making involves taking the same kind of impression that dentists take, only you are the tooth. That is, you sit in a chair (which looks very much like a dentist's chair) and with a bib around your waist, instead of around your neck, an impression is made of your chest, almost exactly the same way as an impression is made of your tooth. It sounded altogether logical when Mr. Lee explained it to me, but I admit that when I was actually seated in the chair, stripped to the waist, and he approached me with a yellow mixing bowl full of a substance that looked like overcooked oatmeal and proceeded to smear it all over my upper body with a plastic spatula, I had my doubts.

The "oatmeal," he had told me earlier, was an alginate which hardens into a rubber consistency the same way it does in the mouth. Needless to say, when it is your chest it doesn't *feel* the same. (At first, it feels repulsive and cold and then, after ten minutes, it feels repulsive and warm.)

Before the substance hardened, Mr. Lee came toward me with another mixing bowl filled with what looked like creamier oatmeal. This was plaster. He then smeared the creamy oatmeal over the lumpy oatmeal and topped it off by wrapping me up in gauze so that, he explained, the substance would keep its shape.

164

When the mess had hardened and I was beginning to wonder how he was planning to get me out of what was now a firm cast, Mr. Lee picked at the top with his fingers, gave it a little pull, and the whole thing peeled off as if it were a banana skin.

"This, you see, is a negative," he said, taking my rubberized configuration into the next room. "Now we fill it with plaster," he shouted so that I could hear him, "and we get a positive, and then we sculpt a replica of the one breast in clay and then we take another cast of that, and *then*," he said, coming back into the room where I was still sitting half naked with the hardened porridge all over my plastic apron, "we make the prosthesis by painting a special mixture of silicone and a catalyst onto the new cast and then it gets hard, we peel it off, fill it up with glycerine, using a little more or a little less glycerine to get the right weight, and we put a backing on it, and that's it!"

"That's really interesting," I said, struggling to get out of the chair.

"Let me help you," he said, and hoisted me down. "Oh—before you get dressed, let's have a look at these." He went over to a cabinet next to the wall and pulled out a few cards of paint samples, mostly tan and some brown.

"What are they for?" I asked.

"That's so we get the right color." He held up one card to the skin of my right breast. "That looks pretty good. . . . It's funny, most women, no matter what the rest of their skin tone is, usually have breasts of this one color." I said yes, that was funny, and wondered what he was doing with the other samples. "Now we match the nipple color," he said, holding up the darker tans next to my nipple. "Hmmm, maybe if we use this and add just a touch of blue." He snapped together the cards. "OK, you can get dressed now."

He went back into the other room while I put my bra and prosthesis and blouse on. When I joined him, he was sitting behind a desk, and I didn't see what was on the desk until he said, "I thought you might like to see what else we do," and then I looked down and there on his green blotter were three ears, two fingers, and a nose.

"Aren't they nice," I said, without moving nearer. "Who are those for?"

"People who have lost other parts of their bodies because of cancer or injuries. I had a woman come in this morning; she was fooling around with one of those power mowers and—*whap!*—there went her third finger."

"Are one of those her—new finger?" I said, trying not to point.

"Oh, no, hers won't be ready for a couple of weeks. . . . I won't have yours until then, either."

I wanted to ask Mr. Lee some more questions, preferably without the digit and features display between us. On the other hand, I didn't want to hurt his feelings by asking him to take them away. I decided to proceed and try to keep my eyes on his

166

face. "How come," I asked him, "made-to-order prostheses are so hard to get? I should think every woman who has had a breast removed would want as exact a replica as she can get."

He shrugged. "Women want them, all right. But they're hard to make. A lot of people have tried and it hasn't worked out. The backs have been irritating or they were too heavy. A million things can go wrong." He smiled. "Terese Lasser has a theory about why there are so few good prostheses. Want to know what it is?"

"Sure," I said.

"She says it's because mastectomies only happen to women. She says if they cut men's testicles off, they would have worked up a great replacement by now."

I laughed. "She's probably right," I said, and then, having forgotten about the display, my eyes moved down to the desk blotter. I looked up at once. "Well, I better get going," I said.

"I'll walk you out to where you can get a taxi," said Mr. Lee, who was really very sweet.

We walked down a long corridor and up to the main floor and out the door. I got into a taxi. "Thanks *very* much," I said. "Good-bye."

"Good-bye," he said, with a nice grin, bending down so that he could see me through the car window. "There's just one thing," he said. "We have had a couple of problems with these things. Uh—if it leaks, just let me know." And the car sped away.

19

AT THE THREE MONTHS' MARK I had an appointment with Dr. Singermann, the first one since he took the bandages off. I was looking forward to the appointment as if it were a date. I was also stiff with fear about what he might find in my right breast.

Negative on both counts. No lump and no thrills. The latter was kind of a letdown—like seeing an old beau who has gotten fat. I was no longer in love with him and he seemed less concerned, medically, about me. Sure, he gave me a thorough examination and he even expressed some interest in my prosthesis hunt. But the fizz was gone. I was an old patient now, in for my trimonthly feel. . . . We had even cleaned up our language.

In the newly laundered version, we did manage a pretty interesting chat, however, mostly about my first visit before the operation. He told me he had lied to me then. He did not think that my chances of having cancer (sorry, a malignancy) were 70/30 or 60/40. He thought they were 97/3. He pulled my card out and read off what he had written on it that day: "duct carcinoma." Cancer. He was that certain that I had it.

He anticipated my next question. "Listen," he said, slamming his hand on the desk, "I regret I told you *that* much. I regret I started in with those numbers at *all*. I've never done that before and I'll never do it again. Smith kept telling me how tough you were. 'She's a news reporter,' he said to me. 'She knows all about it, she can take it.' And look what happened! I started telling you about the different types of surgery and I saw your eyes getting glassy and—"

"Hey, wait a minute," I said, "just because I reacted like a normal human being didn't mean I couldn't take it. Damn it, I *did* take it! So I cried. So what? It was much better that way. It made it *much* easier afterward. But I think you were right not to lay the ninety-seven to three on me. That would have been too rough. . . . By the way, what made you so sure?"

He looked at my card again. " 'Slight puckering when molded.' That means when I squeezed the skin, it puckered slightly. Sometimes there is puckering without molding. But either way, it's a sure sign."

On the way out, I noticed that the secretary who had originally set me up in the hospital was gone. A new girl was in her place. The wastebasket in the examination room brought back memories of my bandage. But even that seemed long ago, like a passage in a novel I had read in school.

That night, when I got home, Erica called. Everything in her life was totally terrible. Because of cuts in the city budget she was sure she wouldn't get tenure at City University, her boyfriend got drunk and hit her, and the kids were driving her crazy. We talked for about a half hour. Erica frets a lot about nothing, but this time things really did sound rotten. We hung up and, as I started cooking dinner, I tried to figure out what she should do about everything and what, if anything, I could do to help. I slid the roast into the oven and, potholder in hand, stood still for a moment in the middle of the kitchen. It occurred to me that I was doing something I hadn't done for a long time. I was worrying about someone else.

At last, I thought.

Work began to interest me again, too, and about six weeks after the operation, a story came up that interested me a lot—on juvenile murderers, the hard-core bad kids. I had only read about them. These were children who were not like children. They showed no remorse or guilt about their crimes, no matter how horrendous—and some of them were very horrendous. And because they were "juveniles," the law could barely touch them. As long as they were underage—younger than eighteen—the most they could get was eighteen months in a detention center, no matter what they had done.

It was a good story, an important story, and I was to do it with someone I especially liked working

170

with: Ira Silverman, an artistic, sensitive, soft-spoken man who also happens to have made the acquaintance of most working gangsters on the East Coast of the United States, including Puerto Rico. I had done a couple of other stories with Ira; they were all worth the fright.

It began to feel like old times again. Almost.

At NBC, at any job, there is bound to be some part of the work that is trivial or boring, some work that does not use the best of one's abilities. For the past decade or so I have had jobs, kept jobs, and like anyone else I've learned to be a good soldier about those parts of the work. No medals, but up in the morning. Most of my "soldiering" at NBC has meant covering a certain kind of "spot" or "hard" news—the straight, no-embellishment kind of story which has never been my cup of tea. In themselves, some spot news stories are riveting, of course. Not for anything would I have missed covering an all-night prison riot in West Virginia a couple of years ago, or the trial of Tony Boyle, whose waxen bird-face I will never forget, or the improbable murder of Governor Sharples of Bermuda. But such stories interested me more as life experiences than as journalistic experiences. These are stories that call for good endurance, on-your-feet thinking, and straight-arrow, factual reporting. It's tough, exciting, and engrossing work, and some correspondents eat it up. But I have always preferred stories called "features" by those who respect them and "soft news" by those who don't. I like them because they allow more time for analysis—and, occasionally, more depth.

Another kind of news assignment which has never given me anything close to pleasure is that nonevent of nonevents, the "stakeout." A stakeout means you are sent off to hang around outside the house or office, or whatever, of someone who doesn't want to see you, and you wait for him (usually not her) to come out, and when he does, you and the forty-seven other reporters who are there ask him a question to which you almost always get a nonanswer.

That's what happens when things work out. When they don't, the person doesn't come out at all, or he sneaks out another entrance, or in some cases he isn't even there. But the reporter on assignment waits and waits and waits and waits and *waits*— outside, usually, where it is inevitably either freezing or broiling—because if he leaves the scene, the other networks, God forbid, might get the nonanswer and not you. The only excuse a reporter has for not being there the moment the person emerges is if he or she has to go to the bathroom. As demanding as the networks are, they do not expect correspondents to rupture their kidneys. Only the cameramen are expected to do that. They can never leave (unless relieved by another) because if the reporter has vanished to pee, at least the cameraman is there to get the stunning shot of the mob of reporters, through whom maybe one can catch sight of the person rushing from the building to an awaiting car. When I leave the scene of a stakeout to pee, I always take as long as possible and hope hard that the person will emerge while I am absent.

I have taken the long way around to say that, one and one-half months after my breast was removed, I was pleased to do the part of my work I enjoyed but felt a growing, firm, unmistakable unsportspersonlike unwillingness to do the rest. Consciously, I hadn't thought much about death since that one awful day, but the mess of numbers and percentages was stored in my head, like roaches in a dark corner. Mostly, I forgot about them, but every time I turned on the light, there they were. If I were going to die fairly soon (unlikely, but not *that* unlikely), I didn't want to spend the time that was left peeling potatoes. Meaning, I didn't want to spend my last weeks, months, or even years attending fires or thrusting microphones in the faces of closed-mouthed (or, for that matter, open-mouthed) figures of public interest. But that was the job, or part of it.

At the same time I was wrestling with all that, I was writing down more and more about what had happened to me, and I knew perfectly well I was not writing for myself. I had never done that and I wasn't about to start. But thoughts of publication made me uneasy, too. I was not writing about felons or John Lennon or Motherhood, but about

173

myself. Personal stuff about myself. Very personal stuff. If I wrote a book, the only way to do it, I knew, was not to hide. But did I really want the world (even the city) to know about my erect nipple? About Arthur? About my shameful self-absorption? I never decided, really. The book just kept coming out. And then it was too late.

So I had a new distraction, more engrossing than shopping for bogus breasts. And it paid. Publication meant an advance. An advance meant enough money to live on. It all added up to a good excuse to leave NBC for a while.

"I hear you've decided to save money on an analyst and write a book," said Wald.

"Yop," I said.

And that was that.

20

PEOPLE ASKED ME if my leaving Arthur had anything to do with the operation. It did, of course, but not in the way they thought. It was not that Arthur was a swine about what had happened to me. He was not. He even rose above the fear that he might be saddled with another invalid like his mother (at least he acted as if he had risen above it). And he never made me feel undesirable or unsexy or anything of that kind. Really, he was the same as ever. We were the same as ever. But that was the problem. Because after the operation, the way we were suddenly scared me.

I put aside what I loved about Arthur. I put aside *that* I loved him. All I could think about now was what was wrong. And, lately, plenty had been wrong. We were fighting more; he was drinking more. I was more critical and sarcastic. We began to nick each other in public, at parties. People thought we were funny. We were. But we didn't feel funny. I thought about it, and the more I thought, the more afraid I got. It was as if there were a slide projector in front of me that kept clicking forward every bad scene we had ever had together: There was the time, only two months before the operation, we were on a vacation in Jamaica and I got sick and wanted a doctor and Arthur thought I was pampering myself and didn't want to call one, until finally I yelled and he called and it turned out I had a 102-degree fever and food poisoning. There was our horrible wedding anniversary last August: I had gotten up at five in the morning to catch a plane for an assignment to run after Nelson Rockefeller somewhere in Maine. I almost lost the story trying to get back in time for Arthur and me to have dinner together. I made it, finally, at about eight thirty, sweaty and exhausted but triumphant. We had a nice dinner, but soon afterward I began to fold. Arthur has never been able to tolerate people folding early. I knew that, but I couldn't help it. I thought he might tolerate it this time. He wouldn't. He got furious. I got furious back. I went to bed. He stayed up and drank. The next morning I sulked and he went off to play tennis. Not a serious scene, but wearing. Nor did we ever resolve scenes like that. They just petered out—until the next one.

All the while David hovered in not-so-distant Philadelphia, waiting for me to quit. But I didn't want to quit. I loved my husband and in his way I knew he loved me. Besides, this much I knew about life: not to expect the moon. Problems are a part of life, I told myself, the way my mother might have told me. Problems are certainly a part of any marriage. You work them out. Or live with them. You don't quit. You don't change husbands like partners at a dance.

But then the music stopped.

And I was frightened. And as the slides kept clicking forward all of those small, bad scenes, I got more frightened. And then I began to think about something that wasn't a scene but a kind of presence between Arthur and me, and that frightened me most of all: other women. Arthur was no major league philanderer, and I felt sure he would never leave me. And mostly all he did was flirt. But that wasn't always all he did. And I thought, If that happens now, I won't be able to handle it. I just won't.

And the fact was, I didn't have to handle it. Because there was David. I wasn't certain I could love David, but I thought I probably could. If I can only work Arthur out of my system, I reasoned, there'll be a space and I will then be able to love David. Anyway, it's worth a try. Because, after all, wasn't David perfect? It wasn't only his hospital vigil or that he wanted to marry me even now, even after what had happened to me. Without all that, he was perfect in himself. First of all, he was monogamous. He said he was, and I believed him. He was attractive and very smart and amusing (not as amusing as Arthur, but so what?), and he was kind and easygoing about everything. And when I stole down to Philadelphia one Wednesday night after

177

work to make sure he didn't mind my missing equipment, I found that he did not. Neither did Arthur, but Arthur just sort of skipped it, while David said a series of perfect things about it, like, "I love you for you, not for your parts." David was a grown-up. He wore suits and ties and he went to an office like somebody's father. Like my father. And he adored me. He said he did and I believed him. Moreover, he said it a lot, in a series of perfect ways, like, "I've never loved anyone in my whole life the way I love you." And he kissed me in the street and in the kitchen (although when we were in his house we didn't go into the kitchen much because there were servants). David was also very, very, very rich.

I had never tied up with a rich man before. I had known some, but they were always boring or arrogant or old (even if they were young) or slick or bad. But not David. He was rich, but none of those other things. It was unbelievable, really. But I decided to believe it. I decided to believe him. And act. Why not? I thought. What better time? There had been an earthquake in my life. Furniture was toppled. Pictures were off the walls. If I was going to do any major life renovations, this was the time to do it, while everything was still a mess. Besides, I thought, I might be dying. What better time to be bold? Do it, I said to myself, do it. Jump. And I did.

Of course, I had not thought through what it would be like to actually gather my things and leave my husband and my home. I did it in the late afternoon, like a thief, while Arthur was at the dentist. I don't think I ever felt so split in two. There was one steely person, full of splendid motor energy, pulling things out of closets; and another porcelain person, cracking quietly in the corner. But the first person toughed it out. She did what had to be done. Her hands were clammy as she packed, laying out clothes in suitcases like bodies in a coffin. But she packed. She packed and she snapped shut the suitcases. And she got out of there.

I was not in good shape when I got to Philadelphia. The New York departure was like surgery and I was still weak from the real surgery four weeks earlier. David was very quiet when I first arrived. He was shaky, too, but I only found that out later. He didn't let me see how shaky he was. That was good of him. Looking back, it was, I suppose, the best of him.

We talked a lot at the beginning. We had a plan. The plan was that I would get a divorce as soon as possible (although I knew from my first few telephone conversations with Arthur that he would not give me an immediate divorce), and we would get married and (not articulated but assumed) we would live happily ever after. You see, I announced to my stunned friends, life *can* be a fairy tale. All it takes is a horror story first. Look at me! Behold the good fortune of your friend, I exulted to Erica,

Pat, Joanna, Leo, et al. All it took was an ounce of flesh. I Suffered and now I'm Getting. See, I *knew* it was a just world. It's like you always said, Mom. Your daughter deserves the best. Only first she had to get the worst.

In my life, I never remember my mother speaking less. She was almost literally dumbstruck. But I could tell what she was thinking. *Was* this a miracle? Or another disaster? I knew just how to convince her. I told her about David, calling up the best cancer man in Philadelphia and making an appointment for me. But that's not all, Mom! Do you know what else this living miracle that your daughter is shacked up with did? He *took* me to the cancer man. This is a man who will take *care* of me, Mother!

The trip to the doctor did make an impression. "I guess something good always comes out of something bad," my mother said in a voice that trembled only slightly. My father thought it was nice that, finally, I was winding up with someone who was Jewish. All Jewish. My friends still didn't know what to think. So I told them.

"I want to marry a grown-up," I thundered at them on the long-distance phone. "My needs have changed, that's all. I *have lost my girlish masochism!* I want someone who will be nice to me. Nice! Good! Caring!"

"But Arthur cares," said Erica in a small voice.

"He *does not,*" I yelled. "He just doesn't want to lose me. That's not the same thing."

"Well," said Erica, "it sort of is."

I didn't call Erica for a week. I didn't want to hear about Arthur caring. I didn't want to hear about Arthur. Every time he called—and at the beginning he called, begging me (unlike him) to come back, once and sometimes twice a day—I cried until my chest heaved so much I was afraid the wound would split open. I stopped answering the phone. That's when the letters began. There was at least one letter a day. And they were worse than the calls!

Dearest . . . I was and am prepared to live with you completely faithfully. Nobody else. That was already part of my psyche when you had the operation. I thought I'd told you that very clearly. I can see how you might have doubted it, and for that I'm deeply sorry. I know the operation shook you to your toes. I can only feel how trembly and uncertain I am from the loss of you to imagine how you must have felt from the loss of a part of you. And I think your decision to depart must have been deeply tied up with the loss of confidence. It would follow, wouldn't it, that even a person as accomplished as you, would, not feeling secure with your husband, gravitate toward an envelope of security, comfort, being taken care of. Naturally, I know nothing of your feelings for the guy. You've never communicated to me any feelings of love for him, but perhaps you only want to protect me from hurt. And yet I get the feeling you hurt, too. . . .

The letter stunned me. Once he stopped calling and began to write I had expected irritation, outrage, even rage. That I could have handled. But not this. Not pain; most of all, not understanding. After the first letter I collapsed.

Then I got up.

Thanks to the God of Geography, my friend Pat Fischer happened to be in temporary residence across the street from David's house. For the entire first week I was in Philadelphia, after David had gone to work in the morning, Pat would ring the bell before the mail came, so that when it did come I wouldn't be alone with the letter. Then, after I had looked at the letter—usually, I couldn't stand to read it—we'd go out for a walk. Those walks were not unlike the early walks up and down the corridors in Beth Israel. But in the hospital I was gayer.

Nor did Society Hill in any way resemble Beth Israel. As neighborhoods go, Society Hill is a good place to be a wreck in. The old streets are as still as heaven, and there is a tidy, insistent grandeur that keeps one from screaming out loud. Pat and I talked continuously during those walks, but I remember much less about what we said to each other than I do about what we saw as we walked: the façades of all those lovely restored houses, with their three-section busybody mirrors at the upstairs windows, their emblems of the different fire companies by the doors, and the old ladies in cloth coats who said "Good morning" and "Good afternoon," depending on when they thought it was.

Later, in May, I got better and it got warmer and

we took longer walks. People were beginning to sit on the benches and on the grass in the parks, faces up to the sun. Sometimes we spread our trenchcoats on the ground and sat for a while, too, half under one of the trees, half in the sun. Pat is a cheerful, plucky little person, so things never got too dour. We even giggled some about our roles: the cuckoo lady in Society Hill (me) and the companion nursie (her).

When the sun dipped behind the buildings of Penn Center, we went back to the house and had tea. Then Pat would go home and I'd write some more and that would keep me together the rest of the day. Then David would come home and we would talk about his work (which I didn't understand but was trying to) and sometimes we'd talk about what I had written that day and we'd have dinner and everything would be fine until the next day and the next letter.

> . . . I think I've changed in a lot of ways, one of which being that I came to see—no matter how I've acted—that I took our *marriage* seriously, our commitment to each other. I still feel like your husband, though it is tough to swallow the fact of your involvement with another's flesh. I wish you wouldn't rush. I wish you'd try to examine the possibility (though I confess he seems to have taken a fatherly role to you) that I'm probably the maturer of the two of us, which ought to count for a good deal, if true. . . .

"If Arthur's letters make you feel that bad,

183

maybe you should go back to him," said Erica. "How can you say that?" I'd shriek. "You *know* how difficult Arthur is. So he's a writer. He knows how to make with the words on paper. How come he never said any of that stuff when we were together? I'm *sure* what I'm doing now is the right thing. . . . David is wonderful."

"Then how come you're so upset by the letters?"

"Erica! It's only *natural* to be upset. Arthur was my husband. I love him. I mean I used to love him. Oh, shit, I can't talk any more. . . ."

And so it went. The truth was I was shocked, horrified, and entirely unprepared for Arthur's show of pain. I felt pain, too, but some of my pain was his. I couldn't tell any longer where his left off and mine started. The pain took a physical turn. My scar began to hurt more. I got stomachaches. I got thinner. Rings fell off my fingers. But I held on. Soon, I said to myself, this will be over and then everything will be all right. I said that to David, too, when he came home in the evening and noticed my less-than-robust appearance. "I know," he said, in his perfect way. "I didn't expect it to be easy." What, I began to wonder, does he really feel? But at that point I didn't really want to know. What if he didn't feel as perfect as he sounded? I wasn't ready for that. I remember how much I looked forward to his coming home each evening, the way I hung over the staircase when I heard the key in the door. First of all, except for Pat, David was virtually

184

all I had in Philadelphia in the way of someone to talk to. And, of course, that wasn't all. Every time he walked in the door, I thought, Here he is: my New Life. Considering what a wreck I was and how taut he was, we had an amazingly nice time during that period. We played records, we played backgammon, we had dinner, we talked. It was pleasant. Low key. Just exactly what my marriage hadn't been. No fights, no stress. Nice talk, nice play, nice sex. Except most of the time I didn't feel that I was really there. But, I reassured myself, soon I will be really here. Soon. Hang on. I hung on. (I always listen to my own orders.) But it didn't feel quite right. It felt more like a new role than a new life.

We had decided it would be a good idea if I didn't go to New York for a while. That was fine with me. The only reason to go to New York at this point was to see Dr. Rumfeld. And, I figured, I could probably "see" him on the phone. He agreed to that. It felt odd, at first, to lie on David's bed at eleven in the morning with Rumfeld's German accent in my ear. But I got used to it. Altogether we had about five sessions on the phone.

"You have had another operation," said Rumfeld. "A separation is like surgery." Ah, that was what I wanted to hear, that my crazy ambivalent feelings were sane. I'd hang up the phone and feel better. Then I'd hear the mail drop through the slot in the front door, and I would walk slowly out of the room and down the stairs and bend down

185

and pick up all the mail, and after putting David's on the foyer table, I'd peel open the back of the envelope that was addressed to me and I'd inhale and read:

. . . I'm terribly afraid that even if you did love me, in the end, and not him, and felt renewed confidence in me (and you), you'd feel so guilty as to not come back even if you wanted to. That you'd tell yourself pain is your lot; that you'd concoct elaborate rationalizations (such as the fact that my being difficult is the reason you left—it surely wasn't the only reason, nor, I think, the main one); that you aren't allowed to be really happy any more; that comfort and security are what you need; that he has nursed you through the touchy part; and so on.

Would you read this letter through a couple of times, please? Try to penetrate what I'm so gummily saying. If you have made a mistake, would you try to see it? Would you try to be brave enough to come back and give me a chance? He'd get along without you.

Just so you don't feel any guiltier about me than you perhaps do, I want you to know that I'm not in perpetual agony any more. I'm surviving and will continue to do so. But I still love you and still long to have you home. I need you, corny as it sounds. I feel almost as though we are two characters in a Greek tragedy, being propelled by forces beyond our control, beyond our conscious will. But our destiny is in our own four hands, yours and mine, and it is completely within our power to put our hands together again. I reach out to you, my adorable, beautiful, lovely wife. I miss desperately your spirit and your body.

A.

P.S. Given the chance, I'd promise to be easier-going, less demanding, less contentious, less insistent on excitements, etc., etc. I wish I could really get sore at you. But I can't. . . .

Fortunately, the mail came before noon, so that I always had more than six hours to pull myself together before David came home.

21

"I AM WORRIED about one thing," began my mother on the phone.

I interrupted her. "Mother, my health is fine. The big cancer guy said I'm fine. I hardly even *think* about the operation." (That was true. Between David and Arthur, I hardly gave cancer a thought— one more reason, it occurred to me much later, for having gone to Philadelphia at all.)

"That's not what I was going to say," said my mother. "I know he's a very nice man, but I just *hope*"—there were implicit "shoulds" or "should nots" in all of my mother's hopes—"that this decision of yours has nothing to do with his money, because your father and I plan to leave you—"

"Mother, it has *nothing* to do with his money. I don't *need* his money. And I don't need *your* money. I earn a lot of money, remember? For God's sake!"

"I was just asking," she said. "Because if it is his money, your father and I plan to—"

"I heard you the first time, Mother. Please!"

But money did have something to do with it, although I didn't think so at the time. Not that I wanted luxuries. I didn't *mind* luxuries, but I didn't covet them. Besides, I was able to afford some on my own without David. Still, I was like a person with a chill, and David's money was like a pile of fleece blankets at the foot of the bed: more than I wanted or needed, but comforting in the extreme to know it was there.

In September, Arthur finally agreed to give me a divorce, so David and I went to Haiti and I got one. It was easy. No children plus no alimony plus plane fare equals instant divorce. It was raining in Haiti. And I cried a lot. In fact, I couldn't stop crying. That was boring of me, but I couldn't help it.

In a way, my divorce was like my wedding—a couple of minutes in a small room in a foreign country with a person with an accent who smiled afterward. The difference was that this time I was alone in the room and *I* didn't smile afterward. "It's natural to feel that way," said the lawyer's secretary, who noticed my quivering lip. I hope so, I thought. I hope so.

Things did change after the divorce. In fact, everything changed. First, Arthur's letters stopped, and I began to feel that he had really left my system. I was totally involved with David and had been since the summer. I felt that I loved David now. And I think he knew that. He said he did and he said how happy it made him. But the funny

189

thing was, he didn't seem as happy as before, when I was giving him grief. And the other funny thing was, he wasn't quite as nice to me as he had been then. The more loving I was toward him, the more withdrawn he got from me, almost sulky. The more commitment I showed about us, the more he began to hedge. He still said all those perfect things about how much he loved me, but he began to say some imperfect things, too. One evening, after dinner, he looked at me and told me he wasn't sure if he loved me. I decided not to make a thing of it. Don't worry, I said. When you live with people, you don't feel crazy about them every minute. It doesn't mean that you don't love them. "Oh," he said.

Well, I thought, he has a right. Look what I put him through. It's his turn now to give me the business.

And he did. He began to complain a lot. He complained about the past—how I had made him suffer —and about the future—how, he feared, I might continue to make him suffer. I can't help the past, I said, but I can do something about the future. What can I do? I asked him. He didn't like my working in New York. Even if I could do stories out of Philadelphia (which I was trying to get NBC to let me do), I'd still have to edit the pieces in New York, and he didn't like that. OK, I said, I'll quit my job. He didn't like my attitude (not positive) about having children. This was not a new attitude of mine.

190

Years before I had written an article for *Look* suggesting that all women were not meant for motherhood (at the time, a radical notion) and that those of us who were not were not necessarily monsters. Fine if you want it, the piece said, but motherhood should be a choice, not an automatic act following marriage. I, myself, was not that *firmly* committed to the idea of not having children, but I certainly leaned in that direction. David knew that. At the same time, I knew that he wanted children. (Although I had always felt that he liked the *idea* of children more than he really would like having them around.) Nevertheless, now he insisted he did, indeed, want children. In fact, he said, he could not live without them. I was somewhat taken aback by the force of this decree, in view of how he knew how I felt about the matter, in view of my being slightly aged for a first child, and in view of the recent wreckage of my body. But he stood firm.

OK, I said, I'll do it. I'll have children. And after thinking about it a few days, I even started liking the idea. It seemed fair enough for him to demand things of me, even difficult things. After all, wasn't he giving me a lot?

But the more I said I'd do what he wanted, the more he seemed to want and the less gracious he seemed to get about what I was willing to do. OK, I thought, so he's not perfect. It's just as well. This way we're even.

Then one day, during a visit to the doctor, things

191

took a very bad turn. It had occurred to me it would be a good idea to check and see how having babies squared with having had cancer. As a rule, David no longer accompanied me on my doctor appointments, but he came along this time.

When I put the question to the doctor, he hesitated. "It's probably OK," he said slowly. "But there is a small risk. During pregnancy there is a rise in the levels of estrogen, and if—*if* there are any cancer cells left in the body, which in your case is unlikely—well, estrogen helps cancer grow."

I felt my stomach turn over like a flapjack. I looked at David. He didn't move.

"But that is a very conservative position," the doctor went on. "Women have gotten pregnant after mastectomies and—"

I interrupted him with the question I'd learned to ask: "If I were your wife, would you let me get pregnant?"

"No," he said, without even a short hesitation.

When we got into the car, I folded my hands in my lap and looked at them and said to David that of course I would be happy to adopt a child. But I understood if that wouldn't do and if he didn't want to marry me any more that it was all right, because I knew how he felt about having his own children. And the only request I had was would he please make up his mind soon. He said he was disappointed, but it was all right. "Are you sure?" "Yes."

For a while the subject didn't come up again. We

both felt too rotten to bring it up. But after a week went by I knew we had to talk about it again. "I know how badly you want children," I said, "and that's made me want them, too. And I want so badly to give you something. But look, if we adopt children, I promise to be a good mother. I will. I *want* to. I'll stop working, I'll—"

David put his head in his hands.

"Oh, dear," I said. "If you really can't bear it, we should end this. Or we should solve it. And then we should feel *good* about how we've solved it. I mean, lots of people adopt children and they love them and it's fine."

He looked at me strangely. His voice was so soft that I wasn't sure at first if I had understood what he'd said. But after a few seconds I understood perfectly. "The doctor didn't say that you *couldn't* have children, did he?"

I stared at him. "Well, that's true. But it sounds risky. It doesn't sound *very* risky. But it's my life. I—I sort of hate to take even a small risk. . . ."

David looked very solemn. "You can be sure I wouldn't ask you to do anything that would risk your life," he said.

David continued to press me about it, though. He had talked again to the doctor, who told him it might not be so unsafe, and he had consulted a top cancer specialist, who said it might be OK in a couple of years, and that there was no evidence to show definitely that it was unsafe. "But that's the point," I

193

said to David while we were in the car one Sunday afternoon. "There are no studies of thirty-nine-year-old women who have had breast cancer and then get pregnant for the first time. The plain fact is those doctors don't know."

"They know that it's a lot safer after two or three years."

"But in three years I'll be forty-two!"

And so it went.

Another time he accused me of being unreasonably frightened. That confused me. I thought, Maybe I am. I no longer knew what to think. About anything.

By this time I was going to New York once in a while, and on one of my trips I went to see Rumfeld. I told him about what was going on. He shook his head. "You were punished by your disease, and now David punishes you for the punishment."

That surprised me. It was very unusual for Rumfeld—for any analyst—to be so baldly critical of one's mate. I found myself defending David. "A lot of men want their own children."

"Yes, but if you cannot have a child, it's not your fault, is it?"

No, I thought, it's not my fault. But it's not his, either. I took a taxi to the station. I was tired, and I had shooting pains in my nonexistent nipple. The four-thirty Metroliner was jammed. I had bought some magazines to read, but I just sat there holding them for a while, staring at the seat in front of me. Then—actually it was an article in one of the magazines that gave me the idea—I thought of a mad and wonderful solution to the baby problem.

I didn't say a word about it to David when I got back; I wanted to make some calls first. I spent almost the entire next day on the telephone. The idea was artifical insemination in reverse. We could find a healthy young girl—a *poor* healthy young girl—who would be willing to get pregnant for money. A lot of money. Then as soon as the baby was born, I'd take over. That would solve everything, I thought. We'd have a baby with David's genes, since that was important to him, and besides that it would be a healthier baby because his or her mother wouldn't have had cancer. I called the doctor first. He thought it was a fine idea and said he would look into it. I called Judy Ramsey, a writer friend who had helped me in the prosthesis hunt. She said it was a great idea and that she would get busy at once to find me a surrogate mother. I called my mother and told her about it, and she said she would write to my cousin who lives in Israel. "Wouldn't it be wonderful to find an Israeli girl? You know the young people there are so poor and so hardworking. And it would be such a good deed." I wasn't sure whom she meant it would be a good deed for, but I didn't pause to ask. Wheels were turning fast now. I was so excited I couldn't wait any longer to tell David. I called him at his office. I blurted everything out and then when I realized he wasn't saying anything back, I stopped.

He sighed.

"You don't like it," I said.

"No," he said, "I don't like it." Neither of us spoke for a few seconds. "Betty," he said, in a certain soft voice I had come to dread, "I want to have children with the woman I love."

I kept up the research anyway, hoping he'd change his mind. He didn't. I started feeling really awful. I hated my deformed and deficient body. I hated what was happening to David and me. We had become foes—each with a position that kept hardening. He really believed that I was manipulating the evidence to get out of doing something I never wanted to do in the first place. After all, had I not happily forsaken any notion of having children long before cancer came into my life? Had I not written an article extolling the joys of nonmotherhood? David also felt that the doctor who said he wouldn't let his wife get pregnant represented one view, no more, no less; and that the other view—that it was all right for me to get pregnant—was just as valid or at least worth considering.

At one point, almost from weariness more than anything else, I thought of giving in. Maybe I'd just do it, get pregnant. The doctor did say his position was "very conservative."

"Hey." I nudged David in bed one night. "Maybe I'll do it."

He turned around and hugged me. "Oh, that would make me so happy," he said. . . .

It would? I thought, watching him fall asleep. It would?

We kept spiraling down. We made a date to get married. We told people. Then he said he had changed his mind; he didn't want to get married that soon. He got cranky. Sex got worse. He still talked nice but I began to see a space between what he said and what he did. I longed for Arthur's lousy public relations.

I longed for Arthur.

The whole thing blew up on a cold, dark Sunday in the middle of December. The night before we had set (another) wedding date, after which, I couldn't help noticing, we both got resoundingly depressed. The next morning we had a brunch to go to in Bala-Cynwyd. That was helpful because, once there, talking to other people made it easier not to talk to each other. But then the brunch was over and we had to leave and we were alone again in the car with this terrible new silence.

When we got back to the house, I took off my coat, shuddered from the coldness that had followed us inside, and hung it up. David had already gone upstairs. As I got nearer to his room, I could hear the click of the television remote control. I hated the sound of that thing. I hated the way David used it. When something was bothering him, he'd pull it out and start clicking pictures on and off . . . sometimes with the sound off. Sometimes he'd do it when he was talking on the phone. He almost always did it when he was talking to his younger sister. I don't know why it bothered me so much. It just seemed gross—like an indolent tic.

He looked up when I came into the room and kept on clicking. Most of the pictures were football games and old movies. Then he clicked it off. I sighed and sat on the foot of the bed. We looked at each other.

"Why don't I feel good about this marriage?" he asked me.

"I don't feel good about it either," I said. "I guess we don't feel good about each other."

"Yes," he said, in a dead voice.

There was some more talk, but it didn't matter. He said he was going out. He left. I packed. My lip trembled. But it wasn't like when I had packed and left New York. It wasn't as bad. Not nearly.

When I got to Penn Station I called Arthur. "I'd —uh—like to have a sort of meeting with you," I said.

"When?" he said.

"Would Wednesday be OK?" (I figured that would give me three days to get myself together.)

"Sure . . . want to tell me what it's about?"

"No," I said, and hung up. Then I leaned my head on my hand, which was still on the receiver, for about ten seconds, closed my eyes, and stayed there without moving at all.

22

IT IS NINE MONTHS since my left breast plus ten axillary lymph nodes were removed from my body. When I took a shower this morning, I shaved under my arms and I could feel, really feel, the razor on the skin of my left underarm. Since that has happened, I keep grabbing myself under the arm, like a baby who has just discovered her genitals.

I am, as my mother would say, my old self. Almost entirely. I am reasonably spirited, but no longer manic. (Or depressive.) I am tearing around again for NBC News the way I used to, which feels normal and good. And, generally, life is moving at much the same pace as it always has: fast.

I am living with my mother now. My father died a couple of months ago—very suddenly, at home, of a heart attack—and I didn't want my mother to be alone. I have not yet absorbed my father's death. When I run across his photograph in a drawer my throat gets tight and lumpy, but I know it hasn't really hit me yet. I'm probably too punchy, still, from everything else. What does hit me is my mother's grief. She is better now, though, than she was at first. It has helped her a lot, she says, to have me here. I guess it has. The apartment is small, so probably in a month or two, or whenever I'm sure she's really all right, I'll move. I'm not sure where.

Arthur and I had our "meeting" that Wednesday night. We had it at the Four Seasons bar; I wanted to go there just because it's pretty. We were both very tender with each other—and very shaky. Arthur was especially shaky. He said I was like someone coming back from the dead. We both cried a little and clutched hands and asked about each other's work and got a little drunk. Since then, we've had some very nice dates (including sleepovers), but we're both being rather cautious about anything more permanent. He is worried, still, that I might go back to David. (I do occasionally hear from David. He writes me letters about how I ruined things by pressuring him too much but says he still loves me and wants to marry me someday.) I want to be sure I don't go back to Arthur as a reaction to David, but for himself, for what we can be together, period—not compared to anyone or anything else. I'm also worried about what kinds of changes there would or wouldn't be between us, if we did try it again. Arthur is concerned about that, too, which in itself is reassuring. Arthur and I are lucky in a way. We have had an uncommon experience. We have both explored our fantasies and found out we like reality better. If I hadn't gone as far as I did with David, I would have thought of him always as that perfect man I didn't marry. And Arthur has since confessed that although having a variety of bedmates was far from boring, it didn't seem to make him feel good in a central way.

It's just as well, I think, that we ended our marriage. Because we did, a new marriage, if there is one, will be a new marriage in every way. We're still the same people, of course, and a lot *wouldn't* change, but that's OK, too. The "perfect" David has made the imperfect Arthur look pretty good. Still, it is clearly best for us, for me, not to do anything for a while. I have, God knows, done enough doing.

As for my body, I am no longer so obsessed with the mirror-mirror-on-the-wall stuff. This is not to say I think I have a keen-looking chest, or that I enjoy being touched or touching myself there. It still repulses me to do that. And I still don't prance around naked. And sometimes when I *am* naked and catch sight of my body's left profile in the mirror and see the narrow, lumpy tube that is my torso, it still makes me swallow hard.

So I swallow hard. There are worse things. Besides, I may get plastic surgery.

Meanwhile, the prosthesis from Michigan hasn't leaked yet and the nipple sticks out nicely. (For three hundred dollars, says Arthur, it *ought* to stick out.) But it is slightly droopier than my other side and it itches slightly and, worst of all, it is such a bother! Gluing it on, pulling it off—or even shoving it in and out of a bra—is like having an extra

201

set of teeth to brush twice a day. It's too much work to do that forever.

The plastic surgery has one of those names: augmentation mammoplasty. Essentially, it involves the same sort of silicone implant that topless dancers get. (Given *my* shape, "topless" suddenly strikes me as a very odd way to describe *those* ladies. Imagine if the drooling butter-and-egg men who go to see those shows got an eyeful of a *real* topless dancer.) Anyway, I hear the surgeons who do this sort of thing can even make nipples, either by grafting skin from the remaining nipple or from the labia minora, of all things, which apparently have the right kind of pigmentation. There is yet another way to get a nipple, but that takes early planning. If one's tumor was originally sufficiently far away, the nipple is sometimes preserved and stored (I am not making this up) in the woman's groin. Dr. Singermann told me about a female surgeon in Montreal who has done this with a number of her patients. She found, however, that when enough time had passed and her patients were able to have the plastic surgery with the nipple replant, they mostly didn't want to bother. (Every time I go to Canada now, or even read something about that country, I think of all those ladies up there walking around with nipples in their groins.)

Even without plastic surgery, I still think I'm pretty, and, in clothes, as sexy as before. I feel sexy in bed, too, but less so than before. I do miss the absent equipment, even if Arthur says he doesn't (and I think he does no matter what he says). And when a strange man gives me a long look on the street or in an airplane or at a party, I do think, What if he knew what I really look like?

I also wonder what it would be like with other men if Arthur and I don't get back together. How would I handle them? It? When would I tell? Obviously it wouldn't be fair to wait until one is between the sheets. Nor is it a good idea, I shouldn't think, to tell a man right *before* one gets in between the sheets, because then, if he doesn't want you any more, he would feel too embarrassed to say so. Probably, then, it's best to tell someone right at the beginning. But how? I could talk about the book, I suppose. That would be a natural way of telling.

But even if a man doesn't mind, how would *I* feel? Maybe all right. I don't really know. If I go back to Arthur I won't ever know. But that's another reason I want to delay a decision about Arthur. I want to be sure I don't go back to him just to avoid the problem of how to tell a new man about the breast I don't have.

As for other people, when I see somebody surveying my chest, instead of feeling bad the way I used to, I just say, "It's the left one." And then I keep on talking, in case they're embarrassed.

Most of these concerns are minor, of course, compared to my worries (not incessant, but daily) about the recurrence of cancer and death. For the most part, I don't think about death directly. I mean I don't sit around trying to imagine it or anything like that. It just crosses my mind, sometimes, like a banner, as if it were one of those advertisements usually, in bed, before I go to sleep. DEATH, says the banner, floating by in a soft wind. It comes at night, hanging from a plane; then it moves along. I don't really *believe* that I will die. It's funny, I *still* don't think it can happen to me. OK, I think, OK, the scythe nicked me. What's-his-name up there made a little mistake. Accidents happen. But that's *it*. I've *had* my accident. Nobody gets hit by a car twice.

Of course, people with cancer usually do. True, people with breast cancer and clear lymph nodes usually don't. But two cancers are still more likely than two car accidents.

Ah, well, I suppose I will breathe easier when three years are up (even two—that's when most recurrences happen), and meanwhile, as they say, you learn to live with it. Sometimes I live better with it than at other times. Minor ailments bring out the worst in me. Ever since I have had cancer, I've become a terrible hypochondriac. The most innocuous physical discomfort elicits, virtually, a fit of terror. I get a headache, I think it's brain cancer. If my foot hurts from a pair of ill-fitting shoes, I am positive I have cancer of the toes.

And I have what may be a permanent kind of anger at my body. My body, which I had always trusted, did betray me, after all. And that is hard to forgive.

204

Fact is, I'm the same car I always was, except now I have a dent in my fender. Of course, I tend to overdramatize some of my (mostly imagined) personality changes. The other day, for example, I was running off at the mouth about one aspect of my new character to my mother. "I'm a lot more impatient now," I said to her earnestly. "I don't want to waste time. I don't want to speak to people I don't want to speak to, or be with people I don't want to be with. I'm less *polite* than I used to be."

"But sweetheart," said my mother gently, "you were *never* polite."

There are some changes, though—not in personality, not in character, as I would sometimes like to think—but in the way I see certain things now, in perspective. This, I know, is trite, but it is also true: When the possibility of death is on one's mind, the problems of life, no matter how great or how niggling, loom less large. When things go well nowadays, I feel as happy as I ever felt before the operation. But the converse has altered remarkably. When things go badly, I definitely suffer less. A personal hurt, a screw-up at work—such things bother me less now, much less.

My raised consciousness about death has somewhat raised my consciousness about life. There is, I find, a recurring jingle in my head:

> Am I doing
> what I'd want to be doing
> if I were dying?

When the answer is no, I don't always act on it, but sometimes I do. More and more I do.

I have made death's acquaintance. And however horrendous and premature that meeting was, I think it will have softened the shock of our eventually living together, whenever that happens. I hope it won't be soon. Because the peek at death has given me some new information about life, all of which has made me better at it than I was before. And, with some more practice, I could get better still. If I don't have a recurrence of cancer and die soon, all I've lost is a breast, and that's not so bad.